Unhealthy or Healthy
EATING
It's Finally Up To You!

BE ENLIGHTENED: THE PSYCHOLOGY OF HOW WE CHOOSE TO EAT

BART P. BILLINGS, Ph.D.

DocUmeant *Publishing*
244 5th Avenue
Suite G-200
NY, NY 10001
646-233-4366
www.DocUmeantPublishing.com

Unhealthy or Healthy Eating—It's Finally up to You!

Be Enlightened: The Psychology of How We Choose to Eat

Published by
DocUmeant Publishing
244 5th Avenue, Suite G-200
NY, NY 10001
Phone: 646-233-4366

Disclaimer: The information and ideas in this book are for educational purposes only. This book is not intended to be a substitute for consulting with an appropriate health care provider. Any changes or additions to your medical or mental health care should be discussed with your physician or mental health provider. The authors and publisher disclaim any liability arising directly or indirectly from this book.

Cover Design by: Sean Strong www.seanstrong.com

Library of Congress Control Number: 2017950432

ISBN#: 978-1-9378-0183-0

Contents

LUNCH OR DINNER

ABOUT THE AUTHOR

Foreword

"You can live a healthier and happier life, if you are careful of;
***what you put in your mouth
and what comes out of your mouth.***"

Bart P Billings, Ph.D.

DR. BART P. BILLINGS is a clinical psychologist who has been in the mental health profession for fifty years. He has worked with all types of patients, including substance abusers, mental hospital patients, physical medicine and rehabilitation patients, patients with weight control problems, etc.

Although Dr. Billings has written and been interviewed on various subjects, such as Vibro-Acoustic Disease (VAD), counseling techniques, psychotherapy treatment programs, Combat Stress, Post-Traumatic Stress Disorder (PTSD), Physical Medicine and Rehabilitation (PM&R) treatment programs, Choice Theory Psychology, Reality Therapy, Traumatic Brain Injuries (TBI), Chronic Traumatic Encephalopathy (CTE), etc., he has for many years stated that general eating habits, exercise, and nutrition play a large role in a person's overall well-being.

Over the last three decades, Dr. Billings has become more and more concerned with health and nutrition issues and has shared with many his concerns about the weight-based problems facing our society that are related to the food we eat and the ways we choose to consume it. Unfortunately most of us grew up learning to favor large quantities of meat, fatty foods, those high in sugar and salt as well as foods that are highly processed. While these behaviors and choices around food have become ingrained in many of us, the good news is that they can also become unlearned and better choices can be made that lead to good health and well-being. An important part of this and foundational to good health is to include more vegetables, fruits and whole grains in your diet. But don't worry! Dr. Billings will not be asking you to eat kale chips and tofu for dinner! Just the opposite, he is going to show you how to take the foods you love and make them healthy! You will never miss the fat, salt and sugar. Promise!

As a former restaurant owner and operator it is not surprising that his kitchen at home includes two stoves, two sinks, an indoor and outdoor pizza oven, and two fully-stocked fridges. One of his favorite hobbies is taking a recipe that is high in calories, salt, sugar, and saturated fats and converting it into a gourmet, healthy meal that has the same look and taste as the original recipe. Dr. Billings also has had experience in a high-end establishment where he was particularly fond of tricking professional chefs by subbing out fatty ingredients for vitamin-packed veggies and lean proteins and not telling them until the meal is over—they never even notice!

Dr. Billings has been invited to speak at grand rounds in integrative medicine programs and has been asked to teach cardiac rehabilitation patients healthy cooking techniques.

While consulting and teaching workshops in various departments at the University of California, Davis, Teaching Hospital at their Medical School, and as a PM&R administrator and psychologist there, Dr. Billings noticed that there were no formal classes for medical students or residents in nutrition beyond basic biochemistry. It is heartening to know that this is beginning to change and more and more medical professionals are becoming aware of the importance of good nutrition in physical and mental health. An example of this changing trend is Tulane Medical School's culinary medicine curriculum, which is now being used by twenty-eight medical schools around the country. This is a good sign of things to come and makes this book a timely addition to the changing health and wellness movement.

Introduction

THIS BOOK WILL EXPLAIN how we have learned what to eat throughout our lifetimes. It will deal with the psychological aspect of what we choose to eat, as well as the effect the media and food industry have on our eating habits and overall physical and mental health.

Everyone has their own history and positive and negative memories growing up, whether they grew up eating fast foods, TV dinners, or home-cooked food. But as will be explained in Chapter 2, human beings have a genetic predisposition to desire fat, salt, and sugar in their diets, even if they grew up eating those things in limited quantities. It should be noted that in societies having limited access to those ingredients, when fast foods containing these ingredients are introduced, the general weight of people increases.[1]

Growing up in Northeastern Pennsylvania, in a family whose ancestry on both sides was Italian, I participated in many traditional eating marathons. My aunt Carmella had a corner grocery

---

1 Popkin, Barry M, Adair, Linda S, and Ng, Shu Wen. "NOW AND THEN: The Global Nutrition Transition: The Pandemic of Obesity in Developing Countries." *Nutrition Reviews* 70.1 (2012): 3–21. Accessed June 13, 2017. https://www.ncbi.nlm.nih.gov/pmc/articles/PMC3257829/

store for over thirty years that sold all types of traditional Italian food. As a youngster, I worked at her store delivering orders and always participated in sampling many of the foods that were sold there. My aunt would always offer me foods such as pepperoni, salami, various types of cheese, chocolate milk, eggnog (when in season), and all kinds of pizzas and pastries. The fruit and vegetable section in the store was secondary to the meats and cheeses.

When I was a senior in high school about to enter college, I graduated from my aunt's corner Banner Food store to a large supermarket for employment. For the next five years, I worked in all the areas of the supermarket: the meat, deli, dairy, grocery and produce departments. Everywhere, there was an opportunity to sample the various foods. Even in the meat department, the store manager, on a slow night, would heat up the package-sealing burners and grill steaks. Most of the time, the foods that were most appealing were from the deli and dairy departments. In the dairy department on Tuesday night, I had to cut large rounds of Romano cheese into wedges and grate them. Tasting a piece seemed like a normal thing to do to be sure it was good enough to sell. Even with gloves on, the next morning in class I had hands that I did not lean on since the odor was stronger than smelling salts. Working in the deli, I became quite good at putting together sandwiches for customers and staff. The sandwiches were piled high with various processed meats and cheeses on Italian bread.

Throughout my childhood, I watched my mother cook for five children, which in itself was a learning experience. But in the family, my father was the gourmet cook of the house. Being the oldest, I watched and helped him prepare some of the meals, both healthy ones (i.e., escarole and beans) and not so healthy (i.e., high-fat pasta sauces with four different meats in the big pot). Many hours were spent making homemade pork sausage with him. As he turned the grinder handle, I held the pork casings that would contain the final sausage mix. It would be nothing for him to make twenty-five pounds of sausage at a time to package up, take to the steel mill where he worked, and sell to his buddies.

My exposure to various types of cooking and eating habits had a direct effect on me and my own children and wife. Later, when moving to California (where I've now have lived for forty-eight years), those early life experiences and the new discoveries in health and nutrition gave me an awareness of foods that are helpful and hurtful. I remember when first coming to California in the late sixties and early seventies, one felt a measure of success by having a freezer in the house with large quantities of beef, pork, and lamb. Cookouts had to feature steaks, burgers, and ribs if they were to be successful. But then in the eighties more and more information came out about nutrition that made an impact on what foods I chose to put into my body. Over time, I learned to make alternate versions of my favorite recipes that were more healthful and just as flavorful.

My change in diet eventually saved my life. Although I always exercised and played sports, I didn't always eat a healthy diet—growing up, I didn't know any better.

Thirteen years ago, a doctor told me that it was a good thing I changed my diet in the eighties and continued exercising. As a result, I was able to overcome much of the damage she found that I did to my body in my childhood and young adult years. The effects of eating foods high in saturated fats, cholesterol, sugar, and salt will eventually catch up with most of us as we age if we don't make changes. But it's good to know that eating correctly and exercising can help overcome damage done years ago. It's similar to a young tree sapling being able to tolerate initially growing in weeds, but as the tree gets older and ages, the weeds choke it and it dies. Let's just figuratively cut the weeds away.

It's funny that for years I thought I was eating really good Italian food in my family home and later what I made myself, based on family recipes. It was not until 1990 when I spent three weeks in Italy, driving from Sicily to Venice and stopping in many cities in between, that I ate *real* Italian food. It's interesting to talk to some people living in the United States of Italian ancestry who visit Italy. I have heard people say that the Italian food in the United States is better than it is in Italy. I asked them to stop and think about what they were saying. They were having *real* Italian food for the first time in Italy and didn't even realize it.

What I realized is that the Italian food made in the United States, even by people who were born in Italy, has been altered to fit our own culture. For example, when in Italy, I observed that meats in pasta sauces were used as a seasoning and not a main ingredient as they are here, since they are more available and cost less in the US.

My uncle once explained to me that when his grandmother came from Italy, she only had a wood-burning stove. As she made sauce on this low-heat stove, she allowed it to sit on the stovetop for hours. Since meat was so plentiful here, she added more of it to the sauce than she would have in Italy. Her children learned the recipe with those new alterations, and that became tradition.

I remember watching my father add sausage, meatballs, cubed beef, and pork chops to pasta sauce that he simmered on the stove for hours. What we thought was the correct way to make Italian pasta sauce was, in fact, changed significantly from the original Italian recipe. As my uncle stated, people with wood-burning stoves, who initially came from Italy, only left the sauce on the stove for extended periods of time due to the fact that the stove was low-heat. When gas stoves and electric stoves became more prevalent, children of Italian ancestry remembered pasta sauces being cooked for hours and didn't take into consideration the type of stove that was used in the initial cooking. As a result, most of the water in the tomatoes evaporated and the sauce was very acidic, as well as fatty from all the various meats. To neutralize the acid, I remember my father adding carrots and celery to absorb the acid and later, when the sauce was completed, he would throw the carrots and celery away. I recall leftover pasta with sauce on it burning small holes in the aluminum foil that covered it, after a day, from the acid of the overcooked tomatoes.

In Italy, I observed cooks making fresh tomato basil sauce in minutes, instead of hours, since this was the way it was intended to be made. I recall occasionally cooking in a five-star Italian restaurant with the chef /owner I knew very well. I watched him add a pound of butter to his fresh tomato basil sauce. He was born in Italy, where this was not customary, and I asked him why he was doing that. He explained that Americans like it that way. So even though customers thought they were ordering a meal low in saturated fats, he added the butter because the chef felt it wouldn't sell unless it was Americanized.

The point is that we in America have gone astray of what our ancestral history and many other cultures have known as healthy, nutritious food. And as a result, we have paid the price with so many of us being overweight, obese, and experiencing life-threatening health problems. This book will begin to unravel how what can only be described as an epidemic came to be and at the same time offer solutions to get back on track to good health.

– 1 –

The Psychology of How We Choose to Eat

THERE ARE MANY PSYCHOLOGICAL theories that can address how people choose to eat, but the one that I find easiest to understand is called Choice Theory Psychology, as developed by Dr. William Glasser, MD.[2]This psychological theory is by no means simplistic, but it is easy to understand.

Once one understands choice theory psychology, not only do eating habits change but the way people relate to others and start living their lives changes. The name itself, "Choice Theory," says it all—most everything people do in their lives is a choice that they make, and the natural consequences of those choices are evident in one's health, family relationships, employment, social relationships, and overall well-being.

Many people I have seen in therapy initially want to put the focus on situations or others for their problems. They avoid assuming responsibility for the behaviors that resulted in their situations in life. Once a person stops blaming others and external situations

2   Glasser, William, MD. *Choice Theory: A New Psychology of Personal Freedom.* New York: HarperCollins, 1999.

1

and assumes responsibility for where he or she is, that's when real change occurs. One of the key aspects of Choice Theory is to get a person to a point where the individual makes a value judgment about his or her past behavior being ineffective and not getting certain desired results. But first they must realize what they really want—not superficial needs, but what psychological needs they want to meet.

What is important to understand is that all human beings have four main higher-level psychological needs that they strive to meet on a daily basis. There is a fifth need that is a more basic physiological need.

First, let's talk about the basic need, which is survival. This need addresses food, clothing, shelter, and procreation. There are countries in the world where people spend most of their time just trying to meet their need to survive and as a result, the higher-level psychological needs are not as important. However, most people in our country have been able to meet this need either on their own or through various social welfare programs.

The higher psychological needs are described as: Love, Power, Freedom, and Fun.

Love

Love can be described as belonging and involvement with others at various intensity levels; a person has many people they interact with and their level of involvement varies with each person. People who experience high levels of involvement with others are generally happy with their lives and enjoy feelings of contentment and fulfillment. On the other hand, people who have lower levels of involvement are usually unhappy with their lives and suffer ongoing psychological pain. In these situations, some people reach out in a negative way to fulfil this need; that's why people join gangs and get involved with addictive drugs and subsequently become addicted people.

When people do not adequately fulfill their need for love, loneliness is a direct result, and loneliness can be seen in many people who overeat. Overeating is a form of addiction, just as strong as using illegal drugs or gambling. Physiologically, when one eats, the body releases glucose (sugars) and other substances into the system that results in pleasurable feelings, but it quickly passes when the food is gone. This type of addiction reminds me of an old movie, *The Loved One*, where the obese, very unhappy woman was feeling so bad that she went into the refrigerator to take out food. While pulling on some food that had frozen together in the freezer, she pulled the refrigerator over on top of herself. Now, picture this person on the floor with a refrigerator on her, causing real physical pain in addition to the initial psychological pain that precipitated this event. What do you think she did to get rid of the physical and mental pain? You probably guessed right: she proceeded to eat out of the refrigerator while it was on top of her. I guess you can say that her addiction to food was an inappropriate and a destructive way to meet her need to feel good.

Like the woman in this movie, when people do not meet their psychological needs in a healthy and constructive way, they attempt to find ways to relieve the psychological pain that it causes.

Meeting needs in a positive fashion creates a sense of active pleasure in which a person can continually enjoy people and experiences throughout his or her life. On the other hand, making negative choices can bring with it fleeting pleasure that subsides when the dysfunctional behavior ends. The woman in *The Loved One* certainly experienced momentary pleasure from eating the food while the refrigerator lay on top of her. However, her negative choices surrounding food resulted in a passive pleasure; she only enjoyed her experience as long as she was eating the food.

So, then, how can one experience authentic, lasting pleasure without resorting to dysfunctional behaviors? Maintaining healthy relationships is one way to cultivate active pleasure in life, as this meets one's need for love and belonging. Taking part in social groups, religious activities, and sports groups can provide active, lasting pleasure as well. The first step is to recognize the difference between pleasures brought about by negative behaviors and then begin to only choose behaviors that fulfill one's need for love and belonging in a healthy, positive way.

Power

The second, higher-level psychological need for power can be described as self-worth, achievement, or simply taking action that draws positive attention to one's self. People meet their need for power through avenues like employment, service clubs, sports, public speaking, politics, etc.

Imagine how powerful a successful performer feels when she sings a song and has an immediate effect on the audience, as evidenced by the applause, yelling, and screaming. Consider the feeling of power a baseball player experiences after hitting a homerun as he listens to the cheering fans while he rounds each base. Not surprisingly, moments such as these result in strong feelings that feed an individual's need for power.

I personally witnessed the power of this need in my own daughter when she was only seven years old. She was performing in a professional regional musical theater in a lead role. There were 3,000 people at the theater. In one scene, she stood alone on center stage with the spotlight on her as she sang a key song in the show. When she finished her song, the audience exploded with applause. After the show, I went backstage and asked my daughter how she felt. She excitedly told me, "My body is tingling all over!" That was the first time in her life in which she experienced that pure power need fulfillment. A year later at another show in which she was featured, she felt that same way again. I explained to her that she experienced those powerful feelings because she was realizing how much of a positive impact she was having on those around her. This understanding not only helped to bolster her sense of self-worth but also resulted in even more exhilaration.

When a businessperson closes a deal or a teacher receives a "thank you" from a student for his or her help, those feelings of power may surface on a smaller scale. However, it is important to note that exceptionally strong feelings of power will only be achieved at special times in one's life. Unfortunately, some people attempt to create that feeling of maximum power each day, especially if they've come across it organically in the past. When they are no longer able to always be in front of large audiences, they try to artificially recreate the feeling with addictive behaviors. Whether it's drugs, food, gambling, or another addiction, the effect is similar to the elevated power need fulfillment they experienced in the past. This explains why wildly successful people sometimes succumb to addictions that ruin their lives; although they have so much to lose, the absence of those powerful feelings causes them to look for ways to fill the void. If it felt good for the performer, athlete or politician to be on their own particular stage, he or she may mistakenly believe that drugs, alcohol, or other addictions can help recreate the same feelings. Unfortunately, no one can expect to feel this powerful all the time, and no substance will change that.

Most people in our society meet their need for power/achievement through their work. That's why when most people meet for the first time, they ask each other what they do for a living. However, there is an important distinction between a career and a job. A career is work that is an extension of who you are—it involves your personality, aptitudes, and passions. On the other hand, a job is something you do to either fill the time or simply to get paid; there is no higher calling and no true personal fulfillment. While a career is need-fulfilling work, a job is transitory and doesn't meet your need for self-worth. Because we tend to fulfill our need for power through work, it is critical for people to find a career that is meaningful—not just a job.

Freedom

The third psychological need is freedom. Many people state that they don't have a choice in their work, living conditions, relationships, etc. Sadly, these people also feel that they *have* to do what they are doing because there are no alternatives. They need to remain in the dysfunctional or painful situation. They can't pursue another line of work. They're stuck living in the house they've been in for years. Fortunately, once people look closely at these statements, it becomes readily apparent that they most often got to the place they are in, good or bad, by the free choices they made in the past.

I once ran training groups (T-groups) for physicians in their residency programs at Pendleton

> **It is very important to meet your need for freedom by choosing to think.**

Navy Hospital. The residents explained that they worked sixty hours a week and had no choice over their hours. They felt like they had no freedom. When they realized that they freely chose to be a physician and part of that choice included a residency requiring excessive hours, they realized that they alone were responsible for where they were at that time. Just knowing that they were freely making a choice gave them an incentive to figure out ways to better handle the stress caused by long hours. They were free to quit, talk with administrators to work out better schedules, develop a more appropriate sleep schedule, etc. They were, in fact, free to make any number of choices to change their circumstances.

I have a friend who was a prisoner of war (POW) in Vietnam for over seven years. He explained that although he was confined in a small cell, he was free to think about what he wanted. He never lost sight of the fact that he was free in his mind to do as he pleased, from sailing to playing golf (or anything else he could imagine). Knowing that no one can deprive you of your freedom to think helped many POWs survive. As documented in my book, *Invisible Scars*, it is interesting to know that no POWs during the Vietnam War committed suicide while in captivity. This was due to their prior military training (i.e., survival, evasion, resistance, and escape), and retaining their cognitive facilities (non-drugged brains) to think and imagine. It is just as striking to note that none of these POWs were given psychiatric medications while held prisoner, such as antidepressants or antipsychotics, which actually impairs your abilities to think clearly and that have a black-box, adverse-effect warning of suicidality, poor judgment and reasoning, anger, hostility, etc.

What the above example illustrates is that it is very important to meet your need for freedom by choosing to think. These thoughts can be positive or destructive. This is one of the reasons why guided imagery is an effective therapeutic tool in many situations.

Fun

The fourth need is fun. It's not surprising to hear from people that they don't have any fun—most people don't even know what fun is. When I explain that fun is learning new information, most of my patients are surprised. Many people associate learning with mandatory schooling. Once they realize that they can choose to learn things that are interesting, "fun" is seen differently. It could be fun learning a new sport, learning a new hobby, learning how to enhance career choices, cooking and learning how to make alternative food dishes with new ingredients, etc.

Having fun also incorporates the first three psychological needs for love, power, and freedom. Fun activities, whether informal classes or other pursuits, involve other people (love and belonging), expand one's skills (power), and provide a choice to be free to perform these activities (freedom).

Effects of the Negative

From the time we are born, we learn ways of meeting the psychological needs described above. We store experiences that meet our needs in our brain's picture album. Almost every meaningful positive experience is stored somewhere in our brain, including holidays with our families, weddings, births, etc. But there are also stored negative experiences. Let's spend a moment looking at negative experiences people may experience, since we hear so much about this in today's media in the form of PTSD. What I described in my last book, *Invisible Scars*, illustrates the types of negative experiences that may be stored in our brains. In this book, I explain that post-traumatic stress (PTS) is a normal reaction for 99 percent of individuals who go into combat. It is simply a normal reaction to being in an abnormal environment. Such things as nightmares, hyper vigilance, restlessness, anxiety, etc. are all normal reactions to abnormal situations. These stress reactions are not only seen in veterans but also in the civilian community when people experience unusual situations such as seeing a car accident or emergency medical situations.

Even if a person doesn't enter combat, it is important to remember that negative experiences are stored within the brain and can be brought to one's consciousness years later. Neglect from one's parents, a failed marriage, financial hardships, and losing a pet are just a few examples of other negative experiences that don't simply disappear with time. The key to dealing with the residual effects of these negative experiences and reactions is realizing that they are normal reactions to abnormal situations, and there are integrative treatment modalities that can deal very effectively with these residual reactions. In other words, there are techniques that help restore healthy ways of thinking and meeting psychological needs in a positive manner, and many of those therapies involve one's choices in life

Choosing to Meet Psychological Needs

Choice Theory Psychology's basic concept is that most human beings can choose how to behave in their lives. These choices, in turn, can affect how well a person meets his or her higher psychological needs for love, power, freedom, and fun. Even in negative situations, it is possible to use Choice Theory to select healthy ways to deal with the residual effects of stress, grief, trauma, etc.

Like a car, the front two wheels determine where we go. The front two wheels here can be seen as thinking and doing. The two back wheels just follow the front wheels' direction. The back two wheels can be seen here as our feelings and physiology. Therefore, the higher four psychological needs—Love, Power, Freedom, and Fun—are the engine that powers the car. The front wheels of thinking and doing let the car know where it should go. The back two wheels of physiology and feelings, in a sense, go along for the ride and are totally responsive to where the two front wheels decide to take the car. So if people want a good, need-fulfilling life, they must pay rigorous attention to what they think and actually do.

Similar to the type of fuel we put in our car, it is also important to point out that the food that fuels our body is of significant importance here as well, since positive nutritional changes can help with mental as well as physical health. Researchers are now showing that healthy dietary changes (i.e., a Mediterranean-style diet) can help improve emotional states.[3]

---

3 Jacka, Felice N., Adrienne O'Neil, Rachelle Opie, Catherine Itsiopoulos, Sue Cotton, Mohammedreza Mohebbi, David Castle, Sarah Dash, Cathrine Mihalopoulos, Mary Lou Chatterton, Laima Brazionis, Olivia M. Dean, Allison M. Hodge, and Michael Berk. "A randomised controlled trial of dietary improvement for adults with major depression (the 'SMILES' trial)." BMC Medicine. January 30, 2017. Accessed June 26, 2017. https://bmc-medicine.biomedcentral.com/articles/10.1186/s12916-017-0791-y.

- 2 -

When We Get Fat, the Food Industry Gets Rich

MY FIRST MAJOR EXPERIENCE with the food industry came as a big surprise. In the past, I had experience selling food in stores, cooking occasionally in a friend's restaurant, preparing foods for large family-and-friends gatherings, and even when going on active duty with the Army, cooking occasionally for the hospital staff I was working with at the time. But I'd never owned a restaurant or spent twelve-hour days on food and its preparation.

It was several years ago that an old friend asked if I could help him with his restaurant expansion. I'd known him for years (he referred to me as his second father), and I decided to help out financially. I figured I'd assist for the first two years, since at the time he had his own television show on the Food Network and had several restaurants that he licensed out to various people. Initially, it was enjoyable stopping by the restaurant, watching the happy customers coming and going, and observing the cooks in the kitchen preparing the food.

My initial excitement about being co-owner of the restaurant only lasted for nine months before the baby was all mine. Nine months into the investment, my partner lost much of what he had achieved and eventually went bankrupt. This left me in sole possession of a restaurant that sold food I wouldn't eat. The restaurant was a barbecue restaurant, serving all the meats that were consistent with barbecue: beef ribs, pork ribs, pulled pork, deep-fried and grilled chicken, various hamburgers, bacon, etc.

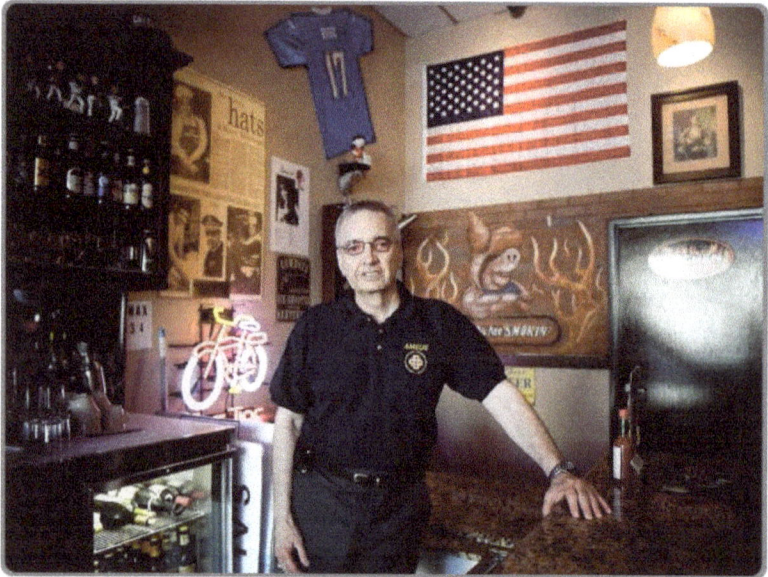

Photo ©2010 Tom Pfingsten, Photographer

Since my forte was healthy nutrition, I decided to implement a heart-healthy section of the menu for self-preservation so I could eat at my own restaurant. My barbecue customers found the additional menu unusual, but their wives did not. It was funny that some of my gentlemen customers complained that coming to the restaurant used to be a refuge from being home, but the new additions (such as wild salmon grilled in lettuce leaves and various salads) meant that suddenly their wives wanted to come with them, and they lost their escape.

The restaurant was also a site for the local Marine base to have promotion parties, staff meetings, and family gatherings. This allowed me to donate free food to the Marines at the local military base on special occasions, such as Christmas parties and special functions. I remember catering for 500 people on base when the US Secretary of Labor visited to discuss training programs.

> "Human beings are evolutionarily wired to prefer fatty and sweet tastes." Lisa Cimperman, Dietician

But the most important lesson I learned at the restaurant was how people are driven to eat large quantities of saturated fats, salt, and sugar—of which barbecued meats have plenty. Dietician Lisa Cimperman claims that "Human beings are evolutionarily wired to prefer fatty and sweet tastes," and in eating barbecued foods, you're looking at saturated fats in the meat and large quantities of sugar and salt in the barbecue sauce.[4] Some of my customers reminded me of cavemen when they came in to eat, especially the bodybuilders and NFL football players. It would not be unusual for some of these people to eat not just one rack of giant beef ribs, but at times two racks and all the trimmings that went along with them, such as French fries, deep-fried hush puppies, etc.

Observing how customers ate at the restaurant reminded me of a medical anthropology course I took in the past. In that course, I recall the professor stating that our early ancestors, thousands of years ago, were basically hunters and gatherers. The men would hunt for meat and the women would gather fruits, vegetables, nuts, and any other plant food that was available. Their eating habits were consistent with their time in history. They did not

---

4 Dealer, Brie Zeltner. "Humans are genetically hard-wired to prefer fat and sugar: Fighting Fat." Cleveland.com. April 04, 2010. Accessed June 13, 2017. http://www.cleveland.com/fighting-fat/index.ssf/2010/04/humans_are_genetically_hard-wired_to_prefer_fat_and_sugar.html.

have regularly scheduled meals, but ate when the food was available. When a wild animal was killed and food was gathered, these early people would gorge themselves on meat and plant foods. The reason they would gorge themselves was because they did not know when their next meal would occur and early on in history, there was no way of preserving food for additional meals. This style of eating is genetically inherent in human beings. At one sitting, they were eating large quantities of animal fat, sugars from various berries and fruits, and salt both in meats and from salt deposits found in nature when they could find it.

When I was in the military, it was required that everyone go through basic training that taught soldiers how to survive on the battlefield. This basic training was considered important for everyone in the military, whether they went on to become a cook, computer programmer, etc. After basic training, they went on to advanced specialty training. Consider the following information your personal basic training for surviving the food industry in our society.

Fats

In general, "fats are nutrients that give you energy . . . [and] have 9 calories in each gram. Fats help in the absorption of fat-soluble vitamins A, D, E, and K."[5] Specifically, fat can be broken down further into saturated fats, trans fats, unsaturated fats, and mono-unsaturated fats. Let's examine each one more closely:

- *Saturated fat*
  "Saturated fat is solid at room temperature, which is why it is also known as 'solid fat.'" This fat occurs naturally in foods originating from animal sources, like meats, cheese, and dairy. Some oils, such as coconut and palm, also contain saturated fat. The recommendation from the

---

5 "Topic Overview." WebMD. Accessed June 13, 2017. http://www.webmd. com/diet/guide/types-of-fats-topic-overview#1.

American Heart Association is to eat no more than 5–6 percent of your daily calories from this type of fat.

- *Trans fat*
  Adding hydrogen to vegetable oil has synthetically produced the majority of trans fats. Trans fat is used in many processed foods to preserve its shelf life and can be found in foods like cookies, chips, and many other snack foods. Doctors recommend avoiding this fat as it increases cholesterol and the risk for heart disease.[6]

- *Unsaturated fat*
  This type of fat is generally a healthier fat to include in your diet, as some unsaturated fats can actually improve cholesterol levels. [7]Unsaturated fats include the following:

  - *Monounsaturated fat*: These fats can lower LDL levels (bad cholesterol) and maintain HDL levels (good cholesterol). Monounsaturated fats are found in foods such as avocados, nuts, and vegetable oils.
  - *Polyunsaturated fat*: These fats are found in plant-based foods and oils and can lower one's LDL levels. This type of fat also includes omega-3 and omega-6 fatty acids:
    - Omega-3 fatty acids can be found in some oils (soybean, canola) and flaxseed, as well as shellfish and fatty fish like tuna, trout, salmon, herring, and mackerel.

---

6 "Trans fat: Avoid this cholesterol double whammy." Mayo Clinic. March 01, 2017. Accessed June 13, 2017. http://www.mayoclinic.org/diseases-conditions/high-blood-cholesterol/in-depth/trans-fat/art-20046114.
7 "Topic Overview." WebMD. Accessed June 13, 2017. http://www.webmd.com/diet/guide/types-of-fats-topic-overview#2.

> Omega-6 fatty acids are found in saffron and soybean oils.[89]

Daily calories per capita by food group, 2010

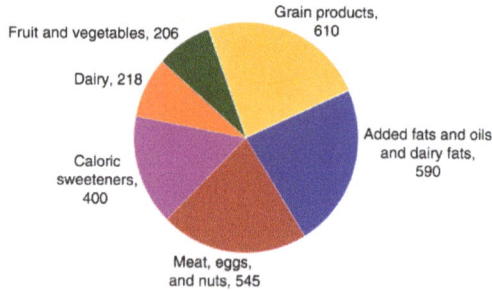

- Grain products, 610
- Fruit and vegetables, 206
- Dairy, 218
- Caloric sweeteners, 400
- Meat, eggs, and nuts, 545
- Added fats and oils and dairy fats, 590

Added fats and oils and caloric sweeteners are added to foods during processing or preparation. They do not include naturally occurring fats and sugars in food (e.g., fats in meat or sugars in fruits).
Source: USDA, Economic Research Service, Loss-Adjusted Food Availability Data.

American diets are out of balance with dietary recommendations
In 2014, Americans consumed more than the recommended share of meat and grains in their diets but less than the recommended share of fruit, dairy, and vegetables

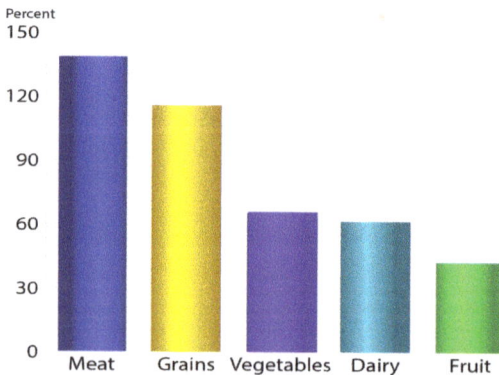

Percent

*Data based on a 2,000-calorie-per-day diet.

Note: Rice and durum flour data were discontinued and thus are not included in the grains group. Food availablity data serve as proxies for food consumption.

Source: Calculated by ERS, USDA, based on data from various sources (see Loss-Adjusted Food Availability Documentation).

Data as of February 2016.

---

8 Ibid.
9 "Dietary fats: Know which types to choose." Mayo Clinic. February 02, 2016. Accessed June 13, 2017. http://www.mayoclinic.org/healthy-lifestyle/nutrition-and-healthy-eating/in-depth/fat/art-20045550.

Salts

Salt is basically sodium chloride, no matter what shape or color it comes in. The Center for Science in the Public Interest states that salt is one of the deadliest ingredients in the US food supply: "While a small amount is safe and necessary for health, the amount of salt in the typical American diet—about a teaspoon and a half a day—is a major cause of high blood pressure, or hypertension."[10]

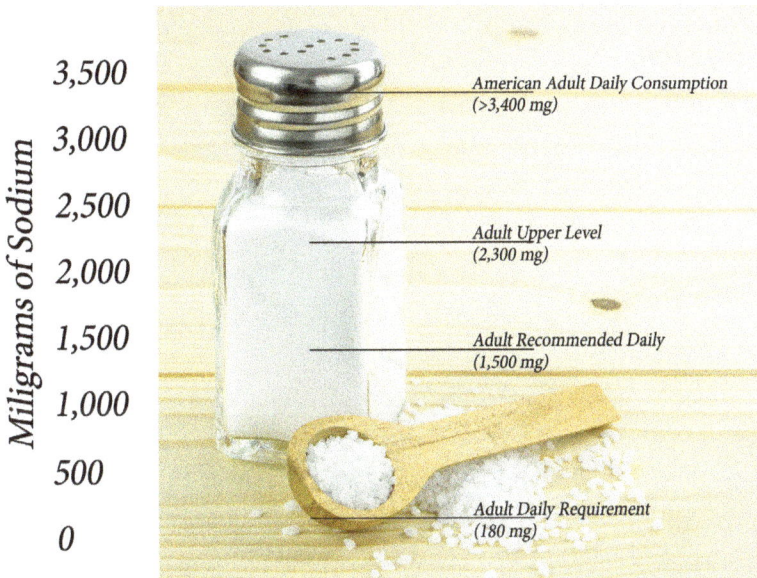

Here are a few other startling facts about a typical American's intake of salt:

- Despite the fact that the *2016-2020 Guidelines for Americans* recommends no more than 2,300 milligrams of salt daily, the average American consumes more than 3,400 milligrams.[11]
- Too much sodium increases one's risk of high blood pressure, and high blood pressure is a major risk factor for

---

10 "Salt." Center for Science in the Public Interest. Accessed June 13, 2017. https://cspinet.org/eating-healthy/ingredients-concern/salt.
11 https://www.cdc.gov/salt/pdfs/sodium_fact_sheet.pdf.

heart disease. Sadly, more than 75 million Americans are putting themselves at risk, since one-third of our population suffers from high blood pressure.[12] [13]

- If Americans reduced their sodium intake to the recommended levels, it would be possible to save between 700,000 and 1.2 million lives over the next ten years.[14]

Sugar Basics

Many Americans love the sweet taste of sugar. However, not all sugar is created equal. Ree added sugars may preserve the food itself, or they may simply be added to improve the flavor or texture of that food. Ice cream, cookies, sodas, pad on to learn more about the different types of sugar, what sugar can do to your body, and what the evolution of corn syrup as a sweetener means for your waistline and health.

> **Excessive salt in your diet puts you at risk of high blood pressure.**
>
> **Added sugars in the blood pose major heath problems as well.**

First, it is important to note that there are two types of sugar: monosaccharides and disaccharides. "Monosaccharides are small enough to be absorbed into the bloodstream" and include fructose, galactose, and glucose.[15] Disaccharides, on the other hand, are combinations of monosaccharides, and they break down once ingested. They include sucrose (table sugar), lactose (milk sugar), and maltose (malt sugar).

Perhaps more important to understand is that there are naturally-occurring sugars—like those found in fruits and dairy

---

12 "High Blood Pressure Frequently Asked Questions (FAQs)." Centers for Disease Control and Prevention. November 30, 2016. Accessed June 13, 2017. https://www.cdc.gov/bloodpressure/faqs.htm.

13 "Sodium and Your Health." Sodium Breakup. Accessed June 13, 2017. https://sodiumbreakup.heart.org/sodium_and_your_health.

14 "Salt." Center for Science in the Public Interest. Accessed June 13, 2017. https://cspinet.org/eating-healthy/ingredients-concern/salt.

15 Accessed June 13, 2017. https://www.accessdata.fda.gov/scripts/InteractiveNutritionFactsLabel/factsheets/Sugars.pdf

products—and added sugars, which are found in many snack foods and sweetened beverages. Thesudding, syrup, pastries, jellies, and jams are just a few examples of foods that contain added sugars.[16] While some naturally-occurring sugars—and even a very small amount of added sugars—in the diet shouldn't pose major problems, the abundance of added sugars becomes concerning, especially when considering the negative health consequences of too much sugar.

What Sugar Does to the Body

In an article on *Nalamag*, the author states that "Sugar raises blood glucose, triggers abnormal insulin surges, and makes us hungry and fat. It also reduces HDL cholesterol (the 'good' kind), skyrockets triglycerides, converts the less-harmful large LDL particles to the much more harmful small LDL particles, and contributes greatly to inflammation in the body. Some scientists even think that sugar is a slow-acting poison."[17]

Other experts agree: "According to Dr. Rachel K. Johnson, lead author of an article published in the American Heart Association journal called *Circulation*, too much sugar not only makes Americans fat, but also is a key culprit in diabetes, high blood pressure, heart disease and stroke. The typical American high sugar diet is also a major factor in the development of cancer and Alzheimer's disease, too."[18]

It's not just the sugar in our food that creates problems, either: sugar-sweetened beverages (SSBs) contribute to health issues as well. In fact, research indicates that there is a "positive correlation

---

16 Ibid.
17 "Affects of Sugar on the Body." Natural Awakenings Southern Louisiana. May 2017. Accessed June 13, 2017. http://www.nalamag.com/Natural-Awakenings-Southern-Louisiana/May-2017/Affects-of-Sugar-on-the-Body/.
18 Kilmer, Kristin. "Everything You Ever Wanted to Know About Sugar." Kristin Kilmer Wellness. April 29, 2012. Accessed June 13, 2017. https://kkwellness.wordpress.com/2012/04/29/218/.

between greater intakes of SSBs and weight gain and obesity in both children and adults."[19] Sadly, many children and adults reach for a soda or other sugary drink without a second thought—and without knowledge of the havoc those SSBs can wreak on their bodies.

Corn Syrup Culprit

A century ago, people didn't have much choice when it came to sweetening their food, as the options were limited to cane sugar, honey, maple syrup, and sorghum. Today, the choices among sweeteners are virtually endless, leading to "significant confusion among American consumers."[20] One major sweetener, corn syrup, has become not only widely used in food and drinks but also a major contributor to weight gain and health issues.

Based on its relatively cheap cost, corn syrup has become manufacturers' favorite go-to sweetener: "Since 1950, corn sweeteners, which are less expensive to produce over sugar cane or sugar beets, has increased 8 times more in our diets."[21] In the past, around the 1970s, the importation of sugar became prohibitively expensive, and to resolve this problem, Japanese scientists discovered a process that could convert cornstarch into a sweetener called high-fructose corn syrup (HFCS). Since the cost of high-fructose corn syrup was significantly less expensive, it replaced the main sweetener in many foods and beverages.

Interestingly, HFCS consumption "increased [more than] 1000% between 1970 and 1990 . . . [mirroring] the rapid increase in

---

19   Malik, Vasanti S., Matthias B. Schulze, and Frank B. Hu. "Intake of sugar-sweetened beverages and weight gain: a systematic review." *The American Journal of Clinical Nutrition.* August 01, 2006. Accessed June 13, 2017. http://ajcn.nutrition.org/content/84/2/274.short.

20   "Everything You Ever Wanted to Know About (25 Types of) Sugar." Small Footprint Family. June 01, 2017. Accessed June 13, 2017. https://www.smallfootprintfamily.com/the-many-different-kinds-of-sugar.

21   Carey, Elea. "High Fructose Corn Syrup vs. Sugar." Healthline. June 16, 2016. Accessed June 13, 2017. http://www.healthline.com/health/high-fructose-corn-syrup-or-sugar#how-bad-is-it3.

obesity."[22] Because high-fructose corn syrup (HFCS) shares a similar composition with sucrose, some research indicates that the body may metabolize this sweetener in the same way the body breaks down sucrose.[23] However, the fact that HFCS constitutes approximately "40% of the caloric sweeteners in the United States"[24] is concerning—and is certainly consistent with significant weight gains over the past several decades. Princeton University psychology Professor Hoebel stated, "Some people have claimed that high fructose corn syrup is no different than other sweeteners, when it comes to weight gain and obesity, but our results make it clear that this isn't true."[25] In addition, the highly-industrialized method of producing it concerns many health experts and environmentalists who are worried about genetic modification and environmental pollution, as well the toxic processing used to create this product.[26]

A report on January 2, 2013 on CBS News stated: "Fructose, a common sugar found in the U.S. diet, may cause changes in the brain that trigger a person to overeat . . . [and] after drinking a fructose beverage, the brain doesn't register the same feeling of

---

22   Bray, George A., Samara Joy Nielsen, and Barry M. Popkin. "Consumption of high-fructose corn syrup in beverages may play a role in the epidemic of obesity." *The American Journal of Clinical Nutrition.* April 01, 2004. Accessed June 13, 2017. http://ajcn.nutrition.org/content/79/4/537.full.

23   Rippe, James M., and Theodore J. Angelopoulos. "Sucrose, High-Fructose Corn Syrup, and Fructose, Their Metabolism and Potential Health Effects: What Do We Really Know?" *Advances in Nutrition.* March 2013. Accessed June 13, 2017. https://www.ncbi.nlm.nih.gov/pmc/articles/PMC3649104/.

24   Ibid.

25   Parker, Hilary. "A sweet problem: Princeton researchers find that high-fructose corn syrup prompts considerably more weight gain." Princeton University. March 22, 2010. Accessed June 13, 2017. https://www.princeton.edu/news/2010/03/22/sweet-problem-princeton-researchers-find-high-fructose-corn-syrup-prompts.

26   Accessed June 13, 2017. http://www.howfoodgrows.com/tag/sap.

being full as it does when simple glucose is consumed, scientists found."[27]

I remember working at the University of California Davis Medical School's Teaching Hospital, seeing patients in the Physical Medicine and Rehabilitation Department. There were all sorts of patients with various impairments, including brain damage.

One day, I had a one o'clock appointment with a brain-injured patient and his parents. The brain damage resulted in this patient losing much of his short-term memory. I remember, during the initial part of the meeting, the patient stated that he was very hungry and couldn't wait to have lunch. His parents indicated that they just came from the restaurant and had eaten a large lunch. But apparently, the brain receptors that determine the amount of food he ate were damaged along with his short-term memory. The patient felt hungry, even though he just ate. This reminds me of what happens when high-fructose corn syrup acts in a similar fashion, temporarily blocking this area of the brain.

So . . . How Much Sugar is OK?

At this point, you may be asking yourself how much sugar is too much. The American Heart Association recommends consuming less than six teaspoons daily for a typical woman and no more than nine teaspoons daily for the average man. Unfortunately, the average American consumes over nineteen teaspoons daily![28] Clearly, we still have a long way to go in reaching the AHA's recommendations.

---

27 CBS/AP. "Fructose changes brain to cause overeating, scientists say." CBS News. January 02, 2013. Accessed June 13, 2017. http://www.cbsnews.com/news/fructose-changes-brain-to-cause-overeating-scientists-say/.
28 Accessed June 13, 2017. https://www.cdc.gov/nchs/data/databriefs/db122.pdf.

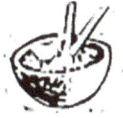

Over the millennia, humans have not lost their tastes for ingredients like salt, sugar, and fat. The problem now is that most Americans eat more than one meal a day. The craving for fats, sugars, and salts is still hardwired into us, but excessive amounts are no longer necessary for survival. In excessive amounts and altered forms, these ingredients can result in severe negative medical consequences. If you stop and think about it, most restaurants and fast food establishments serve significant amount of fats, salts, and sugars in their meals. Eating large volumes of these ingredients on a regular basis is a major contributor to today's obesity and overweight epidemic.

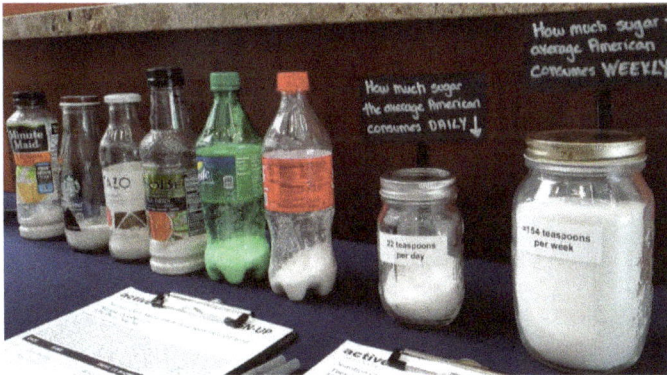

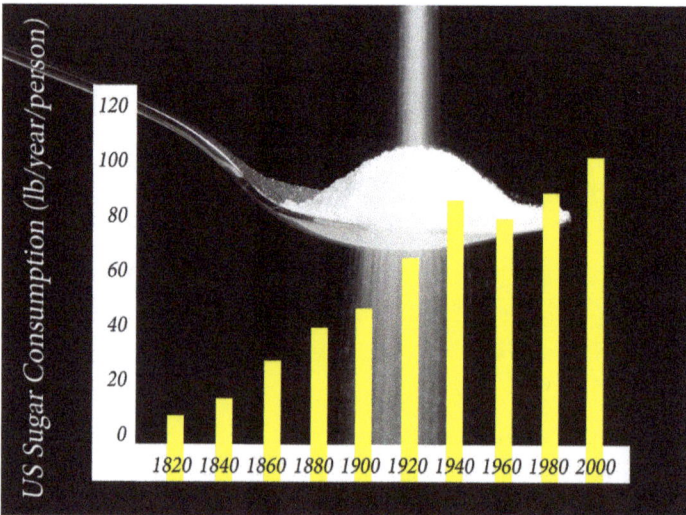

So basically, the food industry knows that people crave fats, sugars, and salts and ensures that those ingredients are in most of their foods. They also know about high-fructose corn syrup causing people to eat more than they need to eat. It's all about making money, without any concern for our society's general physical health. Many of the foods containing these ingredients are consistent with health problems, such as diabetes, heart disease, cancer, obesity, etc.

How one prepares the foods is yet another health concern.

In "Why Deep Fried Foods May Cause Cancer," Dr. Michael Granger stated, "Included in the unhealthy eating pattern was the consumption of deep-fried foods, which have previously been linked to breast cancer, pancreatic cancer, lung cancer, oral and throat cancers, esophageal cancer, and cancer of the voice box." The article also identified higher incidences of prostate cancer.[29]

By heating oils to high temperatures for purposes such as deep-fat frying, you change the molecular structure of the oil, causing

29   Granger, Michael, MD. "Why Deep Fried Foods May Cause Cancer." NutritionFacts.org. July 21, 2015. Accessed June 13, 2017. https://nutrition-facts.org/2015/07/21/why-deep-fried-foods-may-cause-cancer/.

a carcinogenic effect. Later in the book we will discuss healthier oils you can use that will start to burn before their molecular structure changes.

Unfortunately, deep fryers aren't the only hidden danger—grilling foods can cause some of the same types of cancers. An assistant professor of radiation at Harvard Medical School warns readers that "Most of the links between cancer and grilling specifically surround meat, and more accurately meat that is charred or cooked to a high temperature."[30] Later in this book we will describe how to better grill foods to avoid cancer risks.

Clearly one must be cautious of what he or she consumes to live a happy life. As far as eating goes, a person should not consume more calories than what he or she burns in order to maintain a healthy weight. Unfortunately, many Americans are losing this battle, with more than a third of adults in the US considered obese.[31] Consumers, the medical profession, and the government must address this epidemic through intelligent action and education. To paraphrase one of my comments in *Invisible Scars,* knowledge liberates the soul from suffering. In this case, knowledge liberates the body from expanding!

Not only must you increase your knowledge of unhealthy ingredients in the foods you eat, but you must also be aware that some very powerful parties are on a mission to distract and deceive you. Who is this mysterious saboteur?

THE MEDIA.

---

30 Kita, Paul. "Does Grilling Your Food Really Cause Cancer?" *Men's Health.* April 29, 2016.

31 https://www.cdc.gov/obesity/data/adult.html.

U.S. FOOD CONSUMPTION
AS A % OF CALORIES

PLANT FOOD:
Vegetables, Fruits, Legumes,
Nuts & Seeds, Whole Grains
Fiber *is only found in plant foods.*

NOTE: Up to half of this category
may be processed, for example
almonds in candy bars, apples in
apple pies or spinach in frozen
spinach soufflé, and of course these
would not be healthy choices. The
focus should be on whole unprocessed
vegetables, fruits, legumes, nuts and
seeds and whole grains.

ANIMAL FOOD:
Meat, Dairy, Eggs, Fish, Seafood
Cholesterol *is only found in
animal foods. Animal foods are the
PRIMARY source of saturated fat.*

GUIDE TO HEALTHY EATING:
Much easier to understand than the
USDA Food Pyramid, with no food
industry influence.

Eat **LESS** from the animal and processed
food groups and **MORE** whole foods
from the plant food group.

In general, food from the animal and
processed food group contribute to
disease, while **WHOLE** foods from the
plant group contribute to good health.

12%

25%

63%

PROCESSED FOOD:
Added Fats & Oils, Sugars, Refined Grains

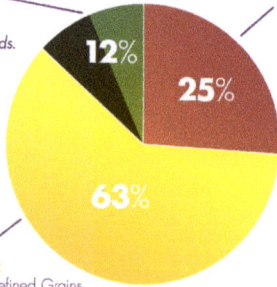

Source: USDA Economic Research Service, 2009, www.ers.usda.gov/publications/EIB33, www.ers.usda.gov/Data/FoodConsumption/FoodGuideIndex.htm#calories
New York Coalition for Healthy School Food • www.healthyschoolfood.org
Special thanks to Joel Fuhrman, MD, author of *Disease Proof Your Child: Feeding Kids Right* • Graphics by MichelleBarda.com
© 2009, New York Coalition for Healthy School Food

- 3 -

How the Media Impacts Our Food

THE MAIN GOAL OF the media is to survive—this requires making money through commercials and advertising from various sponsors, such as pharmaceutical companies, automobile corporations, food companies, and restaurants, to name just a few. Without money from commercials and advertising, these outlets would go out of business.

The website *Statista* is quite valuable in showing how the overall food and beverage industry has spent billions of dollars to influence the general public to purchase their products, which most often may not be good for the general health of consumers. For instance, McDonald's advertising spending ranked fourth in the world, and the food and beverage industry spends a whopping 136.53 *million* dollars every year on advertising! Children aged two to seventeen views anywhere from 476 to 624 candy advertisements each year, in stark contrast to the average 37 to 45 annual views of advertisements for fruits and vegetables.[32]

If that isn't bad enough, companies like Pepsi hire high-profile celebrities to promote their products and pressure consumers to drink or eat what they recommend.

32 Irvine, Victoria. "Topic: Food advertising." Www.statista.com. Accessed June 13, 2017. https://www.statista.com/topics/2223/food-advertising/.

Look at the staggering amounts of money spent on advertising for these food and drink companies:

- Mars: $2.56 million
- PepsiCo: $2.06 million
- Nestle: $2.93 million[33]

Those who are concerned about the extensive distribution of unhealthy food products have suggested there be some type of monitoring of the advertising that is jeopardizing the health of Americans. But like the fight with the tobacco industry, that means taking on an industry that generates trillions of dollars and can afford billions to advertise and defend itself. Fatty, salty, and sugary foods are relatively inexpensive to produce and as a result, money for advertising is plentiful. For example, the cost for the basic ingredients for potato chips and soft drinks is very low; this generates significant profits, even after paying supermarkets shelf-slotting fees and advertising costs.

> Health problems associated with processed foods result in many health problems that the pharmaceutical companies claim to treat.

When we ask ourselves how we can protect the public from this epidemic of unhealthy foods, I think back to the last book I wrote, *Invisible Scars*. In that book I described how the pharmaceutical industry spends billions of dollars promoting brain-altering psychiatric medications. These medications are often ineffective and have significant adverse reactions. In fact, the FDA has mandated "black box" warnings be provided when purchasing these drugs and also when advertising these drugs. I'm sure you've seen at least one antidepressant commercial featuring a happy person prancing around while a background voice rattles off a long list of side effects, including suicide ideation as one.

---

33 http://gaia.adage.com/images/bin/pdf/20151211marketingfactpac kweb.pdf.

In a similar vein, some sort of warning label on certain foods would be an excellent mandatory first step for food advertisers. After all, the food industry works hand-in-glove with the pharmaceutical companies since the health problems associated with processed foods result in many health problems that pharmaceuticals claim to treat.

Imagine if food advertisers were mandated to include warnings while featuring any foods that are consistent with diabetes, heart disease, etc. Warnings such as these could identify the significant amount of fats, sugars, and salt in food products, as well as the associated health risks.

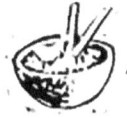

It's important to understand how the food industry tries to influence the least sophisticated individuals in our society: children. First, one must realize that the way the food industry advertises is a highly developed science focused on manipulating parents to purchase their products through children. Including toys and games as part of a child's meal is one method of encouraging children to want to eat that restaurant's foods. And if you stop and think about a popular way fast food restaurants advertise—using mascots that appeal to children—this will help you understand, as an adult, how you are being manipulated through your children to purchase their products.

In addition to advertising, childhood memories can make it difficult to adopt healthy eating patterns. As mentioned in Chapter 1, the associations between certain foods, restaurants, and family time can create positive feelings surrounding particular foods and places—even if those foods aren't healthy. As children grow older, this predisposition to comfort food may influence their adult eating habits. It can even influence the types of food they feed their own children. Many of these unhealthy eating patterns truly pass on from one generation to another, and this can be seen by the continued growing weight and obesity problems in our society.

- 4 -

Why Diets Don't Work—and What Does

A BOOK I READ many years ago written by Bib Schwartz, PhD, first printed in 1982, titled *Diets Don't Work*[34], has been an invaluable resource. I'm sure many other people felt the same way about the book—it's in its fourteenth printing! Dr. Schwartz also wrote a follow-up book titled *Why Diets Still Don't Work*.

Although it has been a few decades since I read the above-mentioned book, its content is still applicable to our world today. The book described the eating habits of naturally thin people, who tend to eat at various times throughout the day. They also eat small amounts of food at no set time; they simply eat out of true hunger. Another point that is important to note is that a person, in order to remain at an appropriate weight for their height and body composition, can't eat more calories than he or she burns if they want to maintain a healthy weight.

I remember Dr. Schwartz talking about an individual who was underweight and wanted to gain weight. To the best my

---

34 Schwartz, Bob. *Diets Don't Work*. Houston, TX: Breakthru Pub., 1996.

recollection, the person he described ate all kinds of fattening foods but just could not gain weight. In order to help him gain weight, he was told to go on a diet, eating even fewer calories than he normally would eat. As a result, his metabolism slowed down. Then, when this individual resumed eating his normal meals, he started to gain weight. This occurred because his body adjusted to the minimal intake of food while he was on a diet and did not speed up when he returned to his regular eating habits.

The body normally slows down its metabolism as a survival technique when food is minimally available. In this situation, the person's brain sensed that food was not plentiful and slowed down his metabolism to increase the chance of survival.

This is the best example that I could find to demonstrate why people who go on diets and initially lose a significant amount of weight most often regain that weight—and more.

For many years in my practice as a psychologist, I had patients who desired to lose weight. The reasons varied from wanting to look better to having health problems as a result of being overweight or obese. I used to joke with my patients that if they followed my advice and didn't lose weight, I would give them a full refund. I never had a patient that came back to me requesting a refund.

My instructions were very easy to understand, but by no means simplistic—losing weight takes dedication and responsibility.

I told them to walk (quickly) at least half an hour a day. I also advised them not to eat any significant food after 5:00 p.m. They could eat small amounts of fruit or yogurt after that time, but no major meals or heavy snacks. In addition, I instructed them to not eat saturated fats (such as those found in red meats), deep-fried foods, and any other pre-made food products with saturated or hydrogenated fats. I explained that they should include in their diet certain wild-caught fish that contained large quantities of omega-3 fats (like wild salmon, sardines, etc.), plenty of vegetables and fruit (preferably organic), and the white meat of organic chicken and turkey. (I did caution them not to eat certain types of fish that were high in mercury content, even if caught in the wild. Also, farmed fish contains certain cancer-causing carcinogens not found in wild-caught fish.)

I explained that this weight loss method was a lifestyle change and not a diet. When people say that it is alright to splurge once in a while, I tell them that recovering alcoholics can't splurge once in a while, since that would be the fastest way of relapsing. When a person wants to change a behavior, whether it is alcoholism, smoking, overeating, or anything else, the more distance they put between themselves and their past bad habit, the less likely they are to slip back when life gets stressful.

> The key to weight loss and control is to consume healthy meals and proportions where you eat fewer calories than you burn.

In all my years of seeing patients for therapy, after following my instructions, I never once had a patient come back and state that he or she continued to gain weight or didn't lose weight. The key for all these patients was to consume healthy meals and proportions where they were eating fewer calories than they were burning.

Eating healthily requires changing some habits. New habits such as using smaller plates, putting your fork down after you consume each bite of food, only putting the food you are going to eat on your plate and storing leftovers in the refrigerator immediately, eating slowly, and chewing food thoroughly all take conscious effort to follow when you're first starting out.

Once those things become habits, though, they'll stick with you for life. My mother-in-law always ate very slowly and was usually the last person to finish her meal. In restaurants, she'd take her time reading through the menu and regarded every meal as an occasion. She lived to nearly 103 and was still in relatively good shape when she passed.

In contrast to this healthy lifestyle, the "7 Habits of Highly Obese People" outlines the patterns of behavior that obese people share:

> **Skipping breakfast raises the obesity risk by 450 percent!**

- They use larger plates, which makes them think they are eating less than they really are.
- They eat while looking at food, which can remind them that there is more food available to eat.
- They eat with maximum efficiency, meaning they use utensils like forks (instead of chopsticks) to eat as much food as quickly as possible.
- They clean their plates.
- They chew less, which relates back to being efficient and quick eaters.
- They dive in; if they are at a buffet, they start serving themselves immediately instead of surveying the options.
- They skip breakfast, raising the obesity risk by 450 percent![35]

Clearly, these "7 Habits" are the complete opposite of the eating patterns among naturally thin people. So now, the question is, how can you avoid bad habits and create healthy ones?

I decided to blend my approach by introducing new behaviors with the knowledge that people have very strong mental images of foods they associate with need-fulfilling behavior, such as love and belonging, achievement, fun, and freedom (as mentioned in Chapter 1). I realize that these pictures of foods that are need-fulfilling cannot be removed from the picture album in someone's brain. Therefore, instead of trying to remove these images that are associated with situations involving family and friends, I decided

---

35 "7 Habits of Highly Obese People." Eat This Not That. January 12, 2015. Accessed June 13, 2017. http://www.eatthis. com/7-habits-highly-obese-people.

that it would be more reasonable to allow the pictures to remain but print them on a different paper. In other words, I wanted to allow the food to look and taste, as much as possible, like what the person originally experienced, but I would use ingredients composed primarily of healthy (Organic) vegetable and animal protein and healthy fats as previously mentioned, instead of unhealthy fats and sugars. The last chapter in this book will have specific recipes to show you how this can be accomplished.

In today's marketplace, we can find many food products that are healthier than products found in previous recipes. A good example would be the various current cheese products that are not made with dairy. Some of the new cheese products are created with almond milk, cashew milk, etc. My daughter lives in the Hollywood area of Los Angeles and frequents a restaurant where all the cheese is made with nondairy ingredients. She tells me that the cheeses in this restaurant actually taste better than the dairy cheese that she used to eat. The line to get into this restaurant is halfway around the block every time she eats there, and this is just one example of how healthy foods can be made in a way that are appealing and do not sacrifice texture and flavor.

Many years ago, I took a medical anthropology course where the professor mentioned that originally only Northern Europeans were genetically able to digest dairy products. He told the story of a famine in a country where the United States decided to provide a high-protein food product to the people there: powdered milk. Because they were not genetically capable of digesting dairy products, they could not utilize the powdered milk in their diet, and mass dysentery ensued.

There are many people in the United States who have difficulty digesting dairy products; hopefully, contemporary restaurants (as mentioned above) and plant-based

> Only 35% of the human population can digest lactose beyond the age of about seven or eight.

cheese manufacturers will satisfy lactose-intolerant people's fond memories from when they were younger and could digest dairy products, with products that are healthier and lactose-free.

Young children almost universally produce lactase and can digest the lactose in their mother's milk. But as they mature, most switch off the lactase gene. Only 35% of the human population can digest lactose beyond the age of about seven or eight. "If you're lactose intolerant and you drink half a pint of milk, you're going to be really ill. Explosive diarrhea — dysentery essentially," says Oliver Craig, an archaeologist at the University of York, UK. "I'm not saying it's lethal, but it's quite unpleasant."[36]

Now you can understand why the pharmaceutical companies produce lactase pills that allow people to ingest a dairy food product that they were never genetically set up to eat. The body has rejected a food that may not be healthy to eat, so modern science has produced a pill to override human genetics.

I recently spoke to a friend that owns a restaurant who mentioned that at a point in his life, he could not tolerate dairy products any longer due to significant GI problems. Even though he had this problem, fond memories of eating large amounts of cheese when he was younger were so strong in him that they led him to eat cheese now.

Along with his fond memories of eating cheese, let's look at another surprising factor that explains why my friend was driven to eat cheese again. A research project reported at http://www.dailymail.co.uk titled "Cheese really is like crack: Study reveals the food triggers the same part of the brain as drugs." states the following: "Cheese is as addictive as drugs because of a chemical called casein. This is found in dairy products and can trigger the

---

36 "Archaeology: The milk revolution." Nature News. Accessed June 13, 2017. http://www.nature.com/news/archaeology-the-milk-revolution-1.13471#b2.

brain's opioid receptors. Opioid receptors are linked to the control of pain, reward and addiction.[37]"

My friend is now proud that he forced himself to overcame this health problem resulting from eating cheese and can now eat cheese again, like when he was younger with no further GI problems. This is particularly interesting because he went from being of average weight to now being obese. It's too bad he did not listen to what his body was trying to tell him.

This is one example of how your body tries to tell you what is good for you and what is bad. There are many other examples, if we look closely, like coughing and feeling nauseous when taking the first drag of a cigarette or cigar, the burn in your throat when drinking strong alcohol (along with getting sick when drinking too much alcohol), and acid reflux that results from eating certain foods and from overeating.

When it comes to successful eating habits, listen to your body. Your body will indicate what food and drink it prefers. Listening to your body will not only allow you to select healthier foods to fuel it but also prevent you from overeating—or eating for emotional reasons that have nothing to do with true hunger.

---

37 http://www.dailymail.co.uk/sciencetech/article-3285478/Cheese-really-like-crack-Study-reveals-food-triggers-brain-drugs.html.

- 5 -

Identifying Healthy (and Unhealthy) Foods

I MENTIONED PREVIOUSLY HOW human beings have psychological needs and physiological predispositions that they strive to satisfy on a daily basis. When describing the psychological needs, I used an example of an automobile having an engine and four tires. The engine is what drives the car to move and the tires take it to where it needs to go. Now I need to mention the fuel that goes into the car that makes the whole system operational. The front wheels of the car being the thinking and doing, the back wheels being the feelings and physiology and the motor being the psychological needs that pushes the vehicle forward. But, without fuel being pumped into the gas tank, or electric current charging batteries in an electric-powered car, the vehicle does not move.

We can use this above analogy to describe the fuel that a human being consumes in the form of food. It is unlikely that a person would put diesel fuel in a gas-operated car or vice versa. It would also be unlikely that an individual would use contaminated fuel to power

75 percent of the US population is overweight and 35 percent are obese.

their vehicle and keep it running smoothly. But many people treat their cars better than they treat their bodies. The fuels they consume in the form of foods and drinks are not always consistent with what a body needs to operate smoothly. Most often when damaging fuel (food) is ingested, the resulting outcome is unwanted medical problems either in the short-term, long-term, or both.

Human beings need basic foods to provide their daily nutritional needs, but as one can see by the fact that 75 percent of the US population is overweight and 35 percent are obese, people do not always appropriately meet their nutritional needs.

The government (authorized by the Clean Air Act) does identify strict requirements for what contaminants are not allowed in the gasoline that goes into our country's cars. There is limited government-required information on food labels, though, which describe general nutritional facts that people should adhere to in our country.

> A good rule of thumb is that if there are long lists of hard-to-recognize ingredients, do not buy the product.

If the gasoline manufacturers do not adhere to specific government regulations for the quality of their fuels, there would be government penalties imposed on them. This is not the case with food companies that do not adhere to government nutritional recommendations in their products.

The government recommendations for daily nutritional needs listed on most food items are as below. Percent of daily values are shown for a 2,000 and 2,500-calorie diet. Your daily values may be higher or lower, depending on your caloric requirements:

Calories	2,000	2,500
Total Fat Less Than	65g	80g

Saturated Fat	20g	25g
Cholesterol	300mg	300mg
Sodium	2,400mg	2,400mg
Total Crbohydrates	300g	375g
Dietary Fiber	25g	30g[38]

It's illuminating to point out that even on a higher-calorie diet, recommended amounts of cholesterol and sodium do not increase.Although the above information exists on most food items purchased in a supermarket, most people are unaware of it or ignore the information. Even with today's smartphones and medical devices, this information on basic nutrition is ignored. Compounding the fact that many people just ignore nutritional data is the fact that when people do try to make sense of it, it's often confusing and misleading.

In the case of not understanding what ingredients are identified on food products, the government needs to step in and ensure that the information is understandable and printed in large type.

Since a significantly large number of people eat at restaurants, it becomes even more difficult to keep track of the food ingredients and amounts of fats, salts, and sugars one ingests. There are some restaurants that offer nutritional data, but the majority of restaurants don't. The old saying "consumer beware" is instrumental to understand when it comes to eating out of the home.

With the Internet and healthy eating food related documentaries on TV, much more information has now become available to the consumer in terms of healthy and unhealthy food. This was not the case when I was growing up in northeastern Pennsylvania.

---

38 Center for Food Safety and Applied Nutrition. "Labeling & Nutrition - Guidance for Industry: A Food Labeling Guide (14. Appendix F: Calculate the Percent Daily Value for the Appropriate Nutrients)." US Food and Drug Administration Home Page. Accessed June 13, 2017. https://www.fda.gov/Food/GuidanceRegulation/GuidanceDocumentsRegulatoryInformation/LabelingNutrition/ucm064928.htm.

As I mentioned previously, it wasn't until the late eighties that I started to pay attention to how I was fueling my body.

If I knew earlier in my life what I know now, there would have been many foods I would not have eaten. Although, in high school I observed the shop teacher demonstrating the acidic effects of cola by pouring a cola on the hood of a car. I watched as the paint was damaged. Throughout the rest of high school and college, I only drank clear soda as a result of this demonstration. So even then I was teachable.

When I was about 12 years old, I have a fond memory of me and a buddy eating pepperoni from my aunt's corner store as we walked to the zoo. At that time in our lives, this was a real treat. Years later, my uncle, who was a professional butcher and owned a grocery store, explained to me that pepperoni did not exist in Italy. According to him, a large meatpacking company created pepperoni in the United States. He told me that when trimming meats, there were large amounts of fats and gristle with only slivers of meat that were discarded. Someone in the company came up with the idea of making money by using the throw-away fat and gristle. The suggestion was made to mix the scraps with paprika, salt, and other spices, put it into a casing, and cure it. They called it "pepperoni."

I recently searched the Internet to determine how accurate my uncle's story was. According to noted food writer and historian John Mariani in his article, "How Italian Food Conquered the World," "Pepperoni is purely an American creation, like Chicken Parmesan." He stated that we do not know its exact origins. It is traditionally made by grinding pork and beef and curing it, using various recipes for the spices.[39] All of the recipes are high in salt and saturated fat. Therefore, my uncle's story of pepperoni's creation is as good as anyone's and sounds logical.

---

39 Mariani, John. "How Italian Food Conquered the World." Accessed June 23, 2017. http://liguriafoods.com/the-history-of-pepperoni/.

Let's take a closer look at pepperoni. The following nutritional information is based on a three-ounce serving:

Calories: 419

Protein: 20%

Fat: 80%

Sodium: 1,479 milligrams

(http://www.livestrong.com/
article/501515-is-pepperoni-good-for-you/)

As we can see, pepperoni is very high in calories. A small serving can easily represent a significant portion of calories allotted for an entire day. It is also very high in fat, with about one third of it being saturated fat—the kind of fat that too many Americans have in their diet. And look at the sodium content—just one serving has almost the daily recommended amount of 1500 milligrams by the American Heart Association.

(https://www.heart.org/idc/groups/heart-public/@wcm/@hcm/
documents/downloadable/ucm_300625.pdf)

What might make this cured meat even more of a health problem is that nitrites are added to the meat to preserve it. The issue is that when nitrites are heated above 266 degrees Fahrenheit, a substance call nitrosamine is created, which causes cancer in animals. (http://www.prevention.com/food/healthy-eating-tips/nitrites-and-nitrates). Nitrosamines have also been linked to diabetes, fatty liver disease, obesity, Parkinson's disease, and Alzheimer's

(http://www.cbc.ca/natureofthings/features/
background-nitrosamines).

The jury is still out as researchers are still undecided as to whether nitrites cause cancer in humans, but until we know for sure, isn't it best just to limit or avoid nitrite-laden foods?

As bad as a stick of pepperoni can be, imagine adding high-fat cheese and carbohydrates found in bread to it. Well, that's one of America's favorite foods—pepperoni pizza!

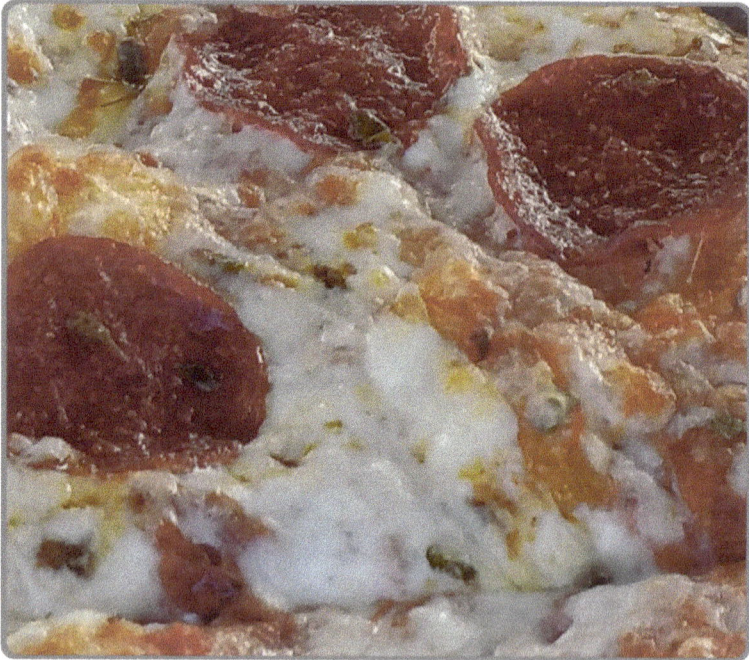

Years ago, I had an opportunity to drive through Italy from Sicily to Venice, with many stops in between. I found that true Italian food contained much less saturated fats and those foods that did were served in limited quantities. The various pizzas I tried in Italy were mostly topped with vegetables, seafood, and minimal meats and cheese. My favorites were eggplants over strips of anchovies, potato pizzas, and fresh basil, garlic, and tomato with olive oil.

I'm not saying that meats in Italy never had large amounts of saturated fats (sopressata isn't exactly fat-free), but fatty foods are eaten in much smaller quantities.

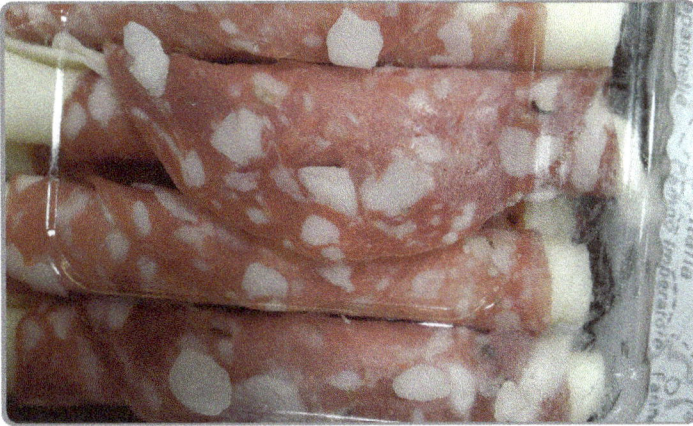

An example of one Italian meat called sopressata

The European Association for the Study of Obesity indicates that the percentage of obese people in Italy is only 10 percent, which is mild compared to the US. The reason may be what I have mentioned earlier; Italians eat less saturated fat. However, that's quickly changing with the youngest generation—36 percent of young boys and 34 percent of young girls are now obese in Italy. An Italian expert in this field and president of the Società Italiana dell'Obesità (SIO), Dr. Sbraccia states that it may be a combination of factors, including increased access to junk food and lack of exercise, which is consistent with the increase in the use of computers and smartphones. Where in the past, when young people were outside playing sports, now this time is taken up with sedentary computer and cell phone activity, which often coincides with mindless snacking. Unfortunately, many areas in the world are in the same boat as the US.[40]

The Institute for Health Metrics and Evaluation states, "Today, 2.1 billion people—nearly 30% of the world's population—are either obese or overweight, according to a new, first-of-its kind analysis of trend data from 188 countries. The rise in global obesity rates over the last three decades has been substantial and widespread,

---

40 "Obesity in Italy." EASO. Accessed June 13, 2017. http://easo.org/media-portal/country-spotlight/obesity-in-italy/.

presenting a major public health epidemic in both the developed and the developing world."[41]

So what in the world is going to do to avert this epidemic?

"Knowledge liberates the soul from suffering" was a quote I used in my book *Invisible Scars*. The Greek philosopher Gorgias, who alluded to this over 2000 years ago, would never have expected it would be applied to the current obesity epidemic. But knowledge through books such as this one and government educational programs appear to be some of the answers. But the general media, who directly create victims in our society through their food advertising and greed to make money at all costs, needs to get on board.

One of the current ways I see the media being positive and educating the public regarding the overweight epidemic is through the production of documentaries explaining proper nutrition and dangers of unhealthy eating.

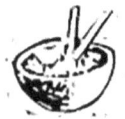

We've talked a lot about what you shouldn't be eating, so what foods are actually *good* for you?

As stated above, a healthy food can become unhealthy if it is eaten to excess. I know vegetarians that are overweight. Moderation is an important aspect of controlling weight gain, but many of the factors mentioned previously may make it difficult to eat moderately. Lifestyle changes and focusing on eating more plant foods is a key factor in changing the direction our world is heading.

---

41 "Nearly one-third of the world's population is obese or overweight, new data show." Institute for Health Metrics and Evaluation. Accessed June 13, 2017. http://www.healthdata.org/news-release/nearly-one-third-world%E2%80%99s-population-obese-or-overweight-new-data-show.

When I talk about lifestyle change, I recall years ago when I was involved with the methadone program in San Francisco. I was in the Army Reserve at the time and had assigned some of my military staff, on their drill weekends, to work in this program. The program worked with individuals who were addicted to heroin. Many were former military from Vietnam. These patients would come in each day to receive their dose of methadone, which is a drug substitute for heroin. On the weekend, their patients would receive a small container with a two-day supply of methadone to hold them over until Monday.

What we discovered was that these individuals would sell their methadone supply on the streets and drink cheap wine to hold them over until Monday's fix. After years of heroin addiction, most of the patients had no jobs and no skills, and they knew that if they could just hold out for a couple of days, they'd get more drugs. There was almost no emphasis on creating a new, healthier life—it was essentially a program to help them change out one drug addiction for another. I tried to convey to the permanent methadone clinic staff was that they needed to work on changing their patients' lifestyles and not just substitute one habit drug for another. When we look at addictive behavior, whether it's illegal drugs or food addiction, we need to consider changing how people can spend their time living differently: exercise, job training, involvement with other people, etc., are all vital.

> **Breaking the hold of addictive behavior needs to take into account how you spend your time.**

The above example explains why, when people have a medical procedure as a result of their bad eating habits, with no lifestyle change, they continue past destructive behavior. An example of what I have stated can be seen in my cousin in Pennsylvania who passed away years ago. He had cardiac bypass surgery, which gave him a second chance in life. Occasionally, I would visit him in his home and watch him eat large quantities of saturated fats, salt, and sugars. His lifestyle had not changed, whether it was his eating or general living situations—he was behaving exactly the same as he did before his surgery. It was only a few years later that he passed away from another heart attack.

I recall another situation at a big church dinner where the main meat course was prime rib. I watched a person cut away fat and then dice it on top of his prime rib. I mentioned to my wife that this person's habit of eating this way could result in a heart attack. He died a short time afterward of just that.

Avoiding Additives

American philosopher Josh Billings stated, "Common sense is instinct and enough of it is genius."

As careful as one may be in watching what they eat, there is another food hazard that takes quite a bit more knowledge to know what to avoid. It has to do with additives, farmed seafood, feed for animals, vegetable and fruit-farming insect sprays, genetic engineering of foods, etc., etc.

To describe in detail all the possible hazards that can cause cancer, diabetes, and other physical illnesses would require a book solely on this subject.

One of the sources of information I recommend you check out is the Truth About Cancer website.[42] Here you will find an informative article titled "Top 10 Cancer Causing Foods: Understanding what Causes Cancer" by Ty Bollinger. I have listed the top ten foods below and if you would like to know more about the relationship of each to cancer you may want to visit their website.

1. Genetically modified foods (GMOs)

2. Microwave popcorn

3. Canned goods

---

42 "Cancer-Causing Foods." Accessed June 13, 2017. https://thetruthaboutcancer.com/cancer-causing-foods-2.

4. Grilled red meat

5. Refined sugar

6. Salted, pickled, and smoked foods

7. Soda and carbonated beverages

8. White flour

9. Farmed fish

10. Hydrogenated oils

In addition to these cancer-causing foods, be very wary of foods that claim to be "light," "diet," or "fat-free," as these items usually use chemicals or unhealthy ingredients to replace natural calories or fat. The result is packaged food items that can produce a variety of health problems.

- 6 -

How to Have a Healthy Pantry

AFTER SPEAKING WITH CHEFS, cooking instructors, and young people, I came to the realization that many young people do not have a decent kitchen set up in their home. Large numbers of young people eat out or order-in food—usually something inexpensive and filling. Foods that meet this description are usually calorie-laden fast foods.

To change this type of eating habit, basic food preparation training is mandatory. When I teach psychological counseling techniques, I tell my class that if you demonstrate involvement, caring, being in the present, and having a real conversation with another person, it's usually a positive experience for all involved. I then use an analogy that it's like cooking: if you use quality olive oil, garlic, and basil, you will generally have a good outcome for just about anything you cook. As they say, *"Keep it simple, stupid."*

So obviously, the food ingredients most people should have in their kitchen cabinet should start with extra-virgin, cold-pressed olive oil. This may sound simple enough, but oils are not always what they pretend to be. It has been discovered that some countries that export olive oil don't necessarily have in the bottle what is stated on the label. Buyers, beware! This misrepresentation occurs with other food ingredients. Therefore, it is critical to shop for food in a credible retail store.

Also, one must be aware of *the containers food comes in*. Overall, I suggest buying food in glass containers if you're not buying fresh or frozen food. Stay away from canned foods due to the probability that they may contain bisphenol (BPA). This ingredient is a plastic that coats the inside of cans in an attempt to keep the foods fresh. Although the FDA states small amounts should not be a problem, human beings are not supposed to eat plastic substances made from crude oil. Bottom line: BPA is poisonous.

I found a terrific piece on this subject from the Seattle Organic Restaurant's newsletter titled, "Five reasons you should avoid canned food; all because they are harmful." According to this article, canned foods are dangerous for the following reasons:

- Bisphenol (BPA): As you already know, you do not want plastics in your food.
- Imported Canned Food: With lower standards when it comes to sanitation and food prep requirements, very little FDA oversight, and 80% fewer nutrients, you will want to avoid canned food from outside the U.S.
- Aluminum Leaks: Canned food poses the risk of aluminum accumulation in the body, and this can lead to memory problems.
- Preservatives: You already know the dangers of salt, and this is a prime preservative in canned foods.
- Low-Level Food Quality: If the produce were truly fresh, then grocers would want to sell it fresh. Think about the risk you're taking when you don't know how fresh—or not—that can of fruit or vegetables may be.

Instead, when possible, purchase fresh foods since "the risk of developing many chronic diseases such as cancer, heart disease, obesity, diabetes, nervous system disorder and Alzheimer's goes down by consuming fresh foods that do not have any packaging." [43]

But even when buying fresh or frozen foods, one should be cautious. A Men's Health article, "Is It Safe to Cook Foods Packaged in Plastic?"[44] states that if using frozen foods, don't cook them in their plastic packaging, since when the plastic is heated, it may release chemicals from the plastic into the food.

Although I don't want this book to be a class in chemistry, one should be aware of harmful chemicals in our environment that may find their way into various foods. An article by Dr. David Carpenter provides information that may be helpful in preserving our health.

> "Reducing one's exposure to synthetic chemicals, i.e., polychlorinated biphenyls (PCB's), can avert potential health problems such as diabetes." Dr. David Carpenter

He states that "Reducing one's exposure to synthetic chemicals, i.e., polychlorinated biphenyls (PCB's), can avert potential health problems such as diabetes. In the late 1970s, approximately 200 chemicals were banned in the US. Many of these chemicals (i.e., PCBs) were used in various products, like flame-retardants in electrical devices, paint and caulking materials, copy paper that did not use carbon paper, and in many plastics. Although these chemicals are not used today, the millions of pounds used in the past remain in the environment in soil and water."[45]

PCBs have been linked to diseases such as cancer and those that suppress the immune system (damage to bones, joints, brain, etc.). Recently, more information reveals that the PCBs also increase the potential for strokes, heart disease, and diabetes.

43   http://www.seattleorganicrestaurants.com/vegan-whole-foods/avoid-canned-food.
44   "Is It Safe to Cook Foods Packaged in Plastic?" *Men's Health.* Accessed June 13, 2017. http://www.menshealth.com/nutrition/is-it-safe-to-cook-packaged-foods.
45   Carpenter, David O., MD. "Beware: New Dangers from the Chemicals All Around Us." *Bottom Line Health* 31, no. 5 (May 2017).

To reduce exposure, one should consider that PCBs are stored in fats found in dairy products, red meats, poultry, and fish. To reduce health risk, one should do whatever is reasonably possible to avoid fats; select cuts of meat with less fat, remove poultry skin, which contains fats (making skinless turkey or chicken breasts a better option.), use non-dairy product substitutes that are lower in fats, etc.

Plain and simple, when possible, purchase fresh foods marked organic and free from pesticides and frozen foods that aren't packaged with material containing BPA. You shouldn't believe there are safe plastics, even if they are labeled as safe. Plastics and foods or beverages shouldn't mix. For more information on this subject, visit the Environmental Working Group at: EWG.org.

Meats—Purchase items that are organically-raised without antibiotics or growth hormones. Grass-fed meats are "rich in inflammation-cooling omega-3 fats . . . [and] also higher in conjugated linoleic acid (CLA), a substance that has been shown to confer a protective property against cancer."[46]

Fish—Purchase fish that is wild-caught. However, one should be selective in choosing what fish to eat, since many fish, even wild-caught, can have excessive amounts of mercury in them, based on their size and how long they live in the water (i.e., swordfish, bluefin tuna, shark, etc.). Some fish I recommend are wild caught salmon (not farmed) from Alaska, wild Halibut from the US, wild-caught Pacific sardines, wild-caught sea bass, wild-caught crab, and lobster from Canada or the US. A good guide for healthy best choices for fish can be found at the Monterey Aquarium Seafood Watch website.[47] And for more information on the dangers of farmed fish, visit https://draxe.com/the-dangers-of-farmed-fish/.

---

46 "Why is Packaged Meat so Dangerous?" Seeker. Accessed June 13, 2017. https://www.seeker.com/why-is-processed-meat-so-dangerous-1770389996.html.

47 http://www.seafoodwatch.org/consumers/seafood-and-your-health.

Try to stay away from imported seafood, since regulations in other countries are not as strict as in the United States. Flash-frozen fish, which is done on the fishing boat, is preferred to buying fish that is not frozen. Unless it's just off the boat, is it difficult to determine how long it has been since fresh fish was originally caught. As a rule for me, I avoid any fish not cooked through, since they harbor parasites that can create health problems. On a side note, the only sushi I eat is baked.

Fresh or frozen fruits and vegetables—Purchasing quality produce is not as easy as it sounds due to genetically modified produce and contaminants from fertilizer and, pesticides. When the Environmental Working Group sampled produce, almost 70 percent of those samples had some form of pesticide residue. Some produce most likely to contain pesticides includes strawberries, spinach, nectarines, apples, peaches, pears, cherries, grapes, celery, sweet bell peppers, and tomatoes.[48]

The best way to reduce the chances of purchasing contaminated produce is to buy organically grown fruits and vegetables, preferably from your local farmers market. However, if you do buy some conventionally grown produce, the following are less likely to be contaminated: sweet corn, avocados, pineapples, cabbage, onions, frozen sweet peas, asparagus, mangos, eggplant, honeydew, kiwi, cantaloupe, cauliflower, and grapefruit.[49]

Food products I generally have in my home:

Note: You should add fresh vegetables and meats to my listed foods below to meet your own individual preferences—use the list below as a starting point only.

Oils—I most often use the following oils. Other oils can be used, but I suggest you research them first for possible unhealthy effects.

---

48 Breyer, Melissa. "Top 12 pesticide-contaminated fruits and vegetables." TreeHugger. May 01, 2017. Accessed June 13, 2017. https://www.treehugger. com/green-food/dirty-dozen-clean15.html.

49 https://www.treehugger.com/green-food/dirty-dozen-clean15.html.

1. Extra-virgin, cold-pressed olive oil. The label should state the harvest month and year, maximum acidity percentage (if you have a problem with acidic foods and digestion, it is recommended you get a maximum acidity level of 0.5 percent), geographical location where it was produced, and certification lot number. Costco has this information on their Kirkland Extra-Virgin Olive Oil bottle. For example, a tablespoon of this extra-virgin olive oil contains: 11 grams (75 percent) of monounsaturated fat (desirable fat), two grams (14 percent) of saturated fat (not generally desirable fat), and one gram (11 percent) of polyunsaturated fat (which in large amounts is not desirable for cooking). For more information on olive oil, visit http://www.marksdailyapple.com/defending-olive-oils-reputation/.[50]

2. Avocado oil is similar to olive oil in the relationship between saturated, polyunsaturated fats, and monounsaturated fats it contains. Avocado oil contains 75 percent of monounsaturated fat, 12 percent of saturated fat, and 13 percent of polyunsaturated fat.[51]

3. Coconut oil contains higher levels of saturated fat (82%) than the above-mentioned oils. But unlike vegetable oils, cold-pressed organic coconut oil is processed differently in the body. Note: In all situations where there are higher amounts of saturated fats in a product, one should check with their physician to determine if using this product will affect their health.

---

50 Sisson, Mark. "Defending Olive Oil's Reputation." Mark's Daily Apple. November 12, 2013. Accessed June 13, 2017. http://www.marksdailyapple.com/defending-olive-oils-reputation/.
51 "9 Evidence-Based Health Benefits of Avocado Oil." Authority Nutrition. June 03, 2017. Accessed June 13, 2017. https://authoritynutrition.com/9-avocado-oil-benefits.

It is important to mention that many vegetable oils, like canola oil, safflower oil, soy oil, and sunflower oil are often processed with chemical solvents and heat, which can cause unhealthy trans fats. Trans fats should be avoided, since the inflammation they cause can increase a person's risk for various diseases (i.e., cancer, diabetes, obesity, heart disease, etc.). Also, unlike animal saturated fat, coconut oil does not store contaminants.

Coconut oil doesn't contain the standard saturated fats, similar to those found in red meats and dairy products. Instead coconut oil contains saturated fats which are medium chain triglycerides (MCTs)—described as fatty acids of medium length. Most of the fatty acids in meat and dairy products are long-chain fatty acids. The medium-chain fatty acids in coconut oil are metabolized differently. They are processed by going directly to the liver from the digestive tract, and used as a quick source of energy or they are turned into ketones. These ketones have therapeutic effects on brain disorders, i.e.dimentia, epilepsy and Alzheimer's.

I personally saw the benefits of coconut oil, first-hand, on my mother-in-law, who lived to be almost 103. When she was 97 years old, we noticed that she was beginning to suffer from dementia. At the time, I read an article stating that the body processes coconut oil differently than other saturated fats.

After checking with her physician for his approval, I gave her two tablespoons a day in her food (one in the AM and one in the PM) of organic, cold-pressed extra virgin coconut oil. Within a few months, she was back to normal cognitive functioning. Now, what really convinced me that the coconut oil was effective was when, after about a year, she started to experience the signs and symptoms of dementia again. I discovered that her roommate, for weeks, forgot to give her the coconut oil. We started her back on it when we discovered this lapse, and she was soon back to being grandma again. She was pretty much alert until her death four years later. After a fall that landed her in a nursing home, the nursing staff there that gave her the coconut oil daily was astonished with the results, to the point that they suggested coconut oil to others in their facility. They even started using it themselves, some in the form of a cream for their skin.

> As we age it becomes more difficult for glucose to enter the brains cells causing them to die.

To explain the incredible results from this oil, we should understand that as people get older, it becomes more difficult for glucose (fuel) to enter the brains cells. When the brain cells don't get the glucose they need to survive, they start to die. Coconut oil has the capacity to get fuel directly into the brain cells. It does this by being broken down into ketones by the liver, and as a result these keytones can cross more easily than glucose into brain cells to provide the necessary sustaining fuel.

If you would like to know more about the benefits of coconut oil here are a couple articles I recommend:

"The Benefits of Coconut Oil for Brain Health", written by Deane Alban. https://bebrainfit.com/coconut-oil-benefits-brain/

"10 Impressive Health Benefits of Coconut Oil"
by Kris Gunnars, BSc. https://authoritynutrition.com/top-10-evidence-based-health-benefits-of-coconut-oil/

Note: The above oils should be bought in small bottles and kept sealed and away from heat and light. This is suggested to prevent them from oxidizing and going rancid. Also, never cook these oils at high heat and never deep fry.

Herbs and spices—I like to keep herbs and spices on hand at all times, in addition to salt and black pepper. But remember, when adding salt or pepper or any other spice to a meal directly from its container, sprinkle it onto your hand if you are not using a measuring utensil, so you can really see how much you are adding. When foods are steaming, this is really important, since steam getting into the container will cake up the seasoning in the bottle and make it spoil.

Similar to the oils, spices should be purchased in small amounts so they don't lose their properties with age. Also they should be stored in a cool, dark place with caps tightened. I suggest that you always use spices from well-known American companies who verify their quality, even if they themselves get them from out of the country. Spices from abroad may harbor pathogens since they don't follow the same safety standards that are in place here in the US. Also, sawdust, pesticides, and other herb fillings have been observed in the past with spices coming from foreign countries. Another safety precaution is to buy whole spices and grind them yourself. This way they are fresher and you know you are getting the real thing. Below is a list of my favorite herbs and spices:

1. Basil (dried or fresh)—As I mentioned previously, if you only have a few spices in the kitchen, basil should be at the top of your list. For more information on basil read Food Facts, "What Is Basil Good For?"[52]

2. Italian Seasoning—A good way to have many spices in one bottle is an Italian seasoning mix. In this mix you will generally find thyme, garlic, marjoram, onion, rosemary, oregano, basil, savory, and sage.

3. Parsley (flakes or fresh)

4. Mrs. Dash (original)

5. Garlic (granulated or peeled and frozen)

6. Onion (granulated or chopped)

7. Chipotle chili powder

8. Cumin

9. Curry powder

10. Oregano

---

52 http://foodfacts.mercola.com/basil.html.

11. Cinnamon

12. Soy sauce (low-salt)

13. Brown mustard (plain or spicy)

Feel free to play around with your spice cabinet; this list is just a good start. All of these can be purchased in glass containers in most stores. If you buy in bulk from a reputable store, be sure to put them in glass containers at home.

Other foods

These foods are perfect to have on hand in a moment's notice. You will also find that you will use many of these ingredients in the recipes from Chapter 7:

Unrefrigerated Food Products

1. Almonds and walnuts (raw or lightly salted)

2. Mixed, unsalted nuts

3. 3. Low-sugar fruit preserves

4. Whole-wheat bread (can be frozen)

5. Almond and peanut butter

6. Organic Chicken and Vegetable broth (low-salt)

7. Non-dairy mayonnaise made with cold-pressed oils

8. White wine (for drinking and cooking)

9. Dried beans (i.e., pinto, lentil, soy, white, etc.)

10. Non-dairy milk (i.e., almond, coconut, soy, rice, or cashew milk)

11. Non-dairy cheese made from almonds, cashews, soy, rice, etc. Can be purchased as block form, sliced, grated, shredded, etc.

12. Worcestershire sauce

13. Honey

14. Sardines (in a glass container)

15. Anchovies (in a glass container)

16. Dates

17. Dried cranberries and raisins with no preservatives

18. Organic brown rice

19. Tomato sauce (in glass container with only organic ingredients)

20. White or yellow onions stored in a cool, dark cabinet

21. Sweet potatoes or yams

22. Tuna fish in water (preferably in glass, if you can find it)

23. Cereals (organic, gluten-free, low-sugar, and free of high-fructose corn syrup)

24. Pasta (preferably whole-wheat, gluten free, also can be made with rice, quinoa, endamame, whole grain, etc.)

25. Red wine

26. Organic popcorn in glass jar

27. Balsamic vinegar that is at least sixteen years old (aged is better and smoother) Note: you can get flavored balsamic, such as raspberry balsamic, chocolate balsamic, etc.

Frozen Foods

1. Spinach (organic)

2. Bell peppers (chopped and organic)

3. Pearl onions (organic)

4. Leeks (sliced and organic)

5. Sweet peas (organic)

6. Broccoli (organic)

7. Non-dairy ice cream (made from almonds, coconut, soy, etc. Low sugar content is preferable)

8. Non-dairy mochi (Japanese ice-cream-like dessert)

9. Chicken gyoza pot stickers

10. Frozen organic fruits

11. Peeled garlic (organic from the US)

12. Frozen wild caught shrimp, scallops, lobster bits, and calamari from US waters (if you are not allergic to shellfish)

13. Chicken strips (organic, cooked from white breast meat)

14. Wild caught salmon, either in steak form or burgers (be careful to get this item with no added ingredients) preferably from Alaska.

15. Wild Alaskan pollock in steak or burger form, with no added ingredients

16. Turkey burgers (organic and with no additives)

17. Chicken breast or burgers (organic, either cooked or uncooked)

Refrigerated Foods

1. Egg whites (organic, get in pint-size containers so they stay fresh)

2. Hummus (organic and in small containers to help stay fresh)

3. Avocado

4. Olives (get a variety in glass bottles)

5. Marinated mushrooms (organic with no chemical preservatives)

6. Soy sauce (low-salt)

7. Non-dairy cheese

8. Dried tomatoes (in glass jar, organic and preservative-free)

9. Chopped Garlic (organic from the US)

10. Non-dairy milk (organic)

11. Non-dairy butter substitute (made with healthy oils)

As previously stated, all of the above-mentioned items are my preferences and can be used as part of a quick meal. This is a good starting point from which to build your own personalized list. And again, all products you use should be organic and free of pesticides or any other substances added to the product.

Cookware: the basics

Now that you have stockpiled your kitchen with healthy, flavorful foods, oils, spices, and herbs, it's time to consider the cookware you will use. The following is a list of cookware that will allow you to cook any recipe in this book, as well as create your own healthy masterpieces:

1. Three ceramic-lined frying pans with lids (six-, ten-, and twelve-inch sizes). I found ceramic-lined frying pans with stainless steel bottoms to be very useful, light, and easy to clean. This is especially important since my original

stainless steel pot and pan set was quite heavy and difficult to handle in the sink when cleaning. One note of caution: when using ceramic pans, never cook on high heat or clean with a coarse pad, as this will eventually ruin the ceramic lining, making it loose its non-stick ability. An advantage of ceramic over Teflon is that ceramic is made without the chemicals PTFE and PFOA, which have a negative effect on the body.

2. For your ceramic pots, be sure to get ceramic or wood utensils so they won't scratch the ceramic. A combination of large cooking spoons, spatulas, and pasta serving spoons are good to have, both in metal and non-scratch materials.

3. A heavy-gauge stainless steel pasta pan with a strainer inside can be used not only for boiling pasta but also for making soups.

4. A hot-air popcorn popper is a must if you like fresh popcorn.

5. A three-quart stockpot made of heavy-gauge stainless steel. This can be used for a variety of foods, as well as for simply boiling water.

6. Toaster

7. Small blender

8. Glass or marble cutting board

9. A quality knife set with knife sharpener

10. Corkscrew for wine with bottle opener

11. Can opener

12. Stainless steel teapot

13. A cutting board made of tempered glass is a great material option for a cutting board, because it's sturdy, treated for thermal shock (resists heat), easy to sanitize in the dishwasher or sink, and sturdy. While it does offer sanitary advantages over wood or plastic boards, one must be aware that, if dropped, it can shatter and that knives will need to be sharpened more often when using it.

14. A microwave oven is great for heating food up quickly or general cooking for most items. But because the cooking can be uneven, be sure to test the food before you eat it to be sure it is cooked through. A great article on microwave cooking can be found on the US Department of Agriculture's Food and Safety Inspection Station.[53] Also, if you want to ensure your microwave does not emit energy outside of the appliance, try this test: place your cell phone in the microwave with the door closed (**DO NOT TURN OVEN ON WHEN PHONE IS INSIDE)** and call your cell phone from another phone. If your phone rings inside the microwave oven, there is a leak in the oven door.

15. Sponges with both a smooth and an abrasive side. To keep sponges from growing bacteria, microwave the sponge (while damp) for one minute on a regular basis.

You can add other cooking utensils as time passes, but the above items are sufficient to do the majority of your cooking. Be careful what else you buy—my cabinets are filled with cookware I very rarely, if ever, use!

---

53 https://www.fsis.usda.gov/shared/PDF/Microwave_Ovens_and_Food_Safety.pdf.

Food Safety

INGREDIENTS AND COOKWARE ISN'T the only thing you need to start cooking. When switching over from processed foods to fresher fare, many new home cooks make simple mistakes that can lead to big problems.

Food safety is of the utmost importance—not keeping things sanitary can lead to some nasty health problems.

This is to certify that

BART P BILLINGS

has met the necessary requirements for
Food Manager Certification.

Exam 6702 Recognized By Conference For Food Protection

FOODHANDLER EDUCATION CERTIFICATE
award to

Dr. Bart Billings C23076

COUNTY OF SAN DIEGO

1 22, 2013

Expires On   Issuing Agent

DIRECTOR OF ENVIRONMENTAL HEALTH

Signature of Cardholder
COUNTY OF SAN DIEGO DEPARTMENT OF ENVIRONMENTAL HEALTH

I obtained the certifications shown above when I owned our restaurant, and as much as I thought I knew, I realized after taking the certification training that I had a lot more to learn.

Again, I am not going to attempt to teach everything I learned, but I'll try to give you some basic kitchen safety information. I recommend that if you can, take a basic food handler's course at your local health department or community college. It could possibly save you from getting food poisoning (or worse).

Many of us have had experiences in our life where we ate something that made us ill. It could have been an allergic reaction to the food itself or the result of eating contaminated food. Years ago, I recall eating chicken from a well-known restaurant chain and getting very ill. Although it was many, many years ago, I never ate their food again. That was one way to avoid getting sick like that again. But there are many other ways to avoid eating bad food, and education is at the top of the list.

> **"Every year the Centers for Disease Control and Prevention receive word of approximately 76 million cases of food poisoning in America."** Forkley.com

According to Forkley.com, "Every year the Centers for Disease Control and Prevention receive word of approximately 76 million cases of food poisoning in America." In this particular article, the author listed the ten foods "most likely to cause food poisoning," and that list includes: chicken, ground beef (and ground chicken), eggs, shellfish (and fish in general), leafy greens, tomatoes, cheese, alfalfa sprouts, deli meats, and berries.[54] Health.com adds four more foods to the list: melons, peanut butter, ice cream, and raw milk.[55]

---

54 Anna in Food on April 2nd. "10 Foods Most Likely to Cause Food Poisoning!" Forkly – Dig In. Accessed June 13, 2017. http://www.forkly. com/food/10-foods-most-likely-to-cause-food-poisoning/.
55 http://www.health.com/health/gallery/0,20310810,00.html.

This doesn't mean you need to cut these foods out of your diet. It does mean that you need to be smart about how and when you consume them.

One of the most important precautions we can take is to be sure we wash our hands thoroughly prior to preparing any food product. It's very important to wash your hands every time you handle a food product before you go to the next food product you are preparing. One example is eggs: the eggshells are a source of bacteria so when handling eggs be sure to wash your hands thoroughly. Bananas and melons are other foods that require washing your hands after handling. There are many others. Also, have a clean work area and clean cutting board.

Cooking foods using a thermometer to ensure they are cooked thoroughly is another important step in keeping them safe for consumption. For meats and fish, you can cut through the surface to the middle to check if it's cooked through. Some important temperatures to know when cooking meat are:

145° F for whole beef, veal, lamb, fresh pork, ham (allowing the meat to cool for 3 minutes before carving or consuming), and fin fish.

160° F for ground beef, veal, pork, lamb, and egg dishes.

165° F for all poultry, including ground chicken and ground turkey, stuffing, leftovers, and casseroles.[56]

When cooking, avoid cross contamination. I often see people using the same spatula to put raw meats or fish on a grill and serving it. This results in cross contamination; bacteria from the uncooked meat or fish are then transferred onto the cooked meat or fish when served. You should always use a separate utensil for putting the uncooked product on the grill. I recall being in a restaurant, watching them grill chicken and the cook doing what I

---

56 "Be Food Safe: Protect Yourself from Food Poisoning." Centers for Disease Control and Prevention. April 18, 2017. Accessed June 19, 2017. https://www.cdc.gov/features/befoodsafe/index.html.

previously described. I immediately left the restaurant. When I owned my own restaurant, I always watched the cooks to make sure this never happened. In the five years I owned the restaurant, we never once got a complaint of food poisoning. Also, don't cut meat on the same board with produce and vice versa. When cleaning cutting boards before storage, you may want to consider adding a small amount of bleach to the water you use to clean the board and then rinse thoroughly. Always wash all produce very well, even those that state they have been previously washed. Scrub the surface of melons with a brush like the one you use on potatoes.

Be aware of what foods are susceptible to contamination based on where they are grown or raised. As mentioned previously, many countries don't have the same safety standards as the US. I personally won't buy foods from certain countries. People should educate themselves as to what countries are safe for food distribution. Also, shop at reliable stores that notify the public of any and all recalls.

Most of all, I suggest that you do more research to get detailed information on food safety—the websites in the footnotes are a great place to start.

I have been telling people for years that home potlucks and buffets in restaurants are the biggest food risks. At a potluck, you don't how dishes were cleaned and if cooked properly. At a restaurant buffet, you don't know the customers handling the serving utensils or if people may have coughed on the food.

Whenever I have a party in my home, I always have a server with gloves and never allow guests to serve themselves. I also put a bottle of hand sanitizer near the table.

I recall my future father-in-law, at my daughter's engagement party, cutting in front of the people in line to eat and trying to serve himself. My server told him it was my orders that no one could serve themselves. It could have been tense when my future father-in-law came to me upset. I explained if he wanted to serve himself, he could wash his hands, put gloves on, and help out as a server. The issue was resolved.

To paraphrase an old saying by Joseph Heller, just because I'm paranoid doesn't mean it's not true. Well maybe we should all be a little paranoid when it comes to food safety, since the Centers for Disease Control estimates that over 70 million people get food poisoning each year—128,000 of those are hospitalized and 3,000 die each year.[57]

The Billings Pot Luck:

If you must have a potluck, I suggest that you contact a restaurant near your home that you trust that has good food and sanitary conditions with an A rating from the health department on the window. If you have twenty couples attending your party, call the restaurant and identify up to twenty items you want to serve. Some orders can be half orders where two people each bring a half order.

By doing this, everyone makes a choice of what they want to buy and pays generally the same price, with you having the assurance that the food was prepared correctly in a sanitary health-department-inspected kitchen.

Now you have the responsibility as a host to ensure the food is kept warm on heat trays or chilled on ice. Eating promptly always helps and when outside, keep food chilled with ice and in the shade, especially foods that spoil quickly, such as mayonnaise-based salads like potato salad and coleslaw.

For more information on food handling, I suggest you turn to the Illinois Department of Public Health, which has great

---

57 "Estimates of Foodborne Illness in the United States." Centers for Disease Control and Prevention. August 19, 2016. Accessed June 18, 2017. https://www.cdc.gov/foodborneburden/index.html.

information on appropriate cooking, holding, and storage temperatures for food.[58]

With plenty of cookware, healthful ingredients, herbs and spices on hand, and basic knowledge of food handling safety, you're ready to start cooking some (healthy) gourmet meals. Read on to the next chapter for some of my favorite recipes.

58 "Critical Temperatures for Food Service." Food Safety Fact Sheet - Critical Temperatures for Food Service. Accessed June 18, 2017. http://www.idph.state.il.us/about/fdd/fdd_fs_foodservice.htm.

- 8 -

Your Favorite Comfort Foods— *Upgraded*

SO MANY OF MY therapy patients were people who made choices in their lives that resulted in emotional anguish. My job was to help those people learn how to develop an alternative way of dealing with life's stressors. Prior to therapy, they typically had one way—and one way only—to deal with their situations. Sadly, their way of dealing with issues was usually ineffective, and they had difficulty seeing alternative choices. In working with these patients, I determined that they needed to learn to apply this alternative thinking mindset to their own lives.

What I found effective for these people was to teach them how to develop **alternative thinking habits**. I wanted to teach them to develop a thought process like a radio scanner; you scan many stations, and the station that has the most powerful signal is where the scan stops. I would ask them to practice identifying five different ways of doing everyday tasks. For example, before leaving my office, I would ask them to consider five different ways they could get home: they could take the freeway, take the back streets, call their spouse and meet for dinner and then go home, take a cab or

Uber, or call a friend and be picked up. Five ways to get dinner could include: make it from scratch, order home delivery, stop and pick it up, stop at a friend's house and eat there, or visit a restaurant.

The five ways don't necessarily have to make perfect sense; it was the thought process that was the purpose for this exercise.

> Cook food with healthier ingredients, while keeping it—as much as possible—the way it looked and tasted.

Throughout my career, I held many management positions where I used this same approach in dealing with problems. When I was a hospital commanding officer in the US Army, I told my staff I would not discuss a problem with them unless they had formulated at least three ways of resolving it. Now, they didn't need to be reasonable ways! I just needed to know that my staff was taking the time and energy to look for solutions.

I remember three nurses who were on their way to see me regarding a problem. I watched them walking down the long hallway to my office. As they approached my door, they shook their heads, turned around, and walked away. Later, I asked what happened. They said that they knew I wouldn't speak with them unless they had three alternatives to solve their problem. By the time they reached my door, they came up with a good solution and no longer needed to meet with me!

I have learned to use this same alternative thinking process when cooking. As I explained in Chapter 1, we have foods that we grew up with that are associated with positive relationships and experiences in our lives. We store pictures of those comfort foods in our memories. I don't want to attempt to remove this positive picture, but just change the paper it is printed on. In other words, let's cook the food with healthier ingredients but keep it as much as possible, the way it looked and tasted. Also we may be able to add positive pictures of new food experiences that are associated with current experiences.

This chapter will give you some recipes for healthy versions of my favorite comfort foods. Once you get used to experimenting with better ingredients, you can create better versions of your own favorite foods!

Recipes *(Many can be made in one pan.)*

The recipes below will help you learn to make fantastic dishes using healthy ingredients. When using these recipes, always remember that you should keep your options open—add your own favorite herbs, spices, and healthy add-ins to truly personalize the dish. *Also substituting plant based food products for any animal based ingredient is always an option. And always remember that when you can, use organic foods, free of pesticides, antibiotics etc. and other added artificial ingredients.*

In the same way, feel free to use more or less of the ingredients listed below to meet your desired tastes. When you think about alternative cooking methods, consider two or three different ways you can make each recipe with healthy and safe ingredients. The recipes below will give you a general idea about how you can make meals that are tasty and healthy to eat. You can build from these examples.

Always remember the Old Italian proverb, "What the eye cannot admire the heart cannot desire." In other words, always make your food appealing to the eye, and always eat on a cloth placemat (or paper mat, if cloth is not available). When eating in a restaurant with a hard tabletop, I always ask for another napkin so I can put my plate on it. Every meal should be special and not just routine. That way, you get into the habit of eating special, quality food.

Also, smell the food while cooking. Fan the steam toward you with your hand. You can not only enjoy the aroma but also gauge if you need to add more seasonings. I find that most of the time, if it smells good, it tastes good.

WARNING: All stoves have different heat sources and burner tops, so the cooking temperatures listed below should be adjusted to your heat source.

Breakfast

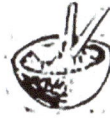

Let's start with something very quick and simple.

Toast with Toppings

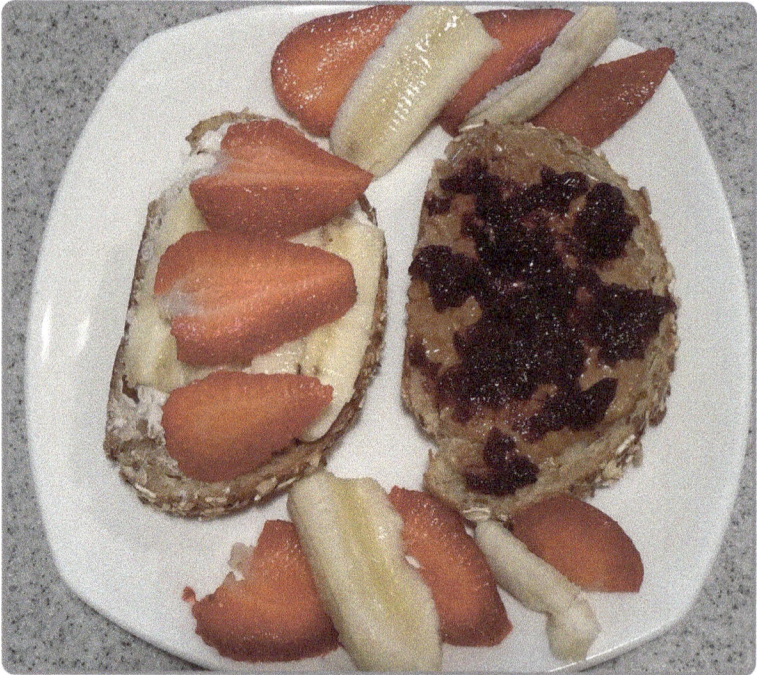

INGREDIENTS

1 tbsp. of almond butter

2 tsp. of blueberry preserves (low-sugar)

1 thick slice of whole-wheat or whole grain bread (or gluten-free)

PREPARATION

Lightly toast the bread and spread on the almond butter and blueberry preserves.

Alternative toppings for toast can include: non-dairy cream cheese with fresh blueberries or bananas sliced lengthwise and sliced strawberries with a dab of non-dairy sour cream on top if desired.

Ingredients replaced: butter, white bread, peanut butter, dairy-based cream cheese, dairy-based sour cream, and high-fructose corn syrup in preserves.

Egg-White Frittata
(Leftovers can be refrigerated and reheated the following day)

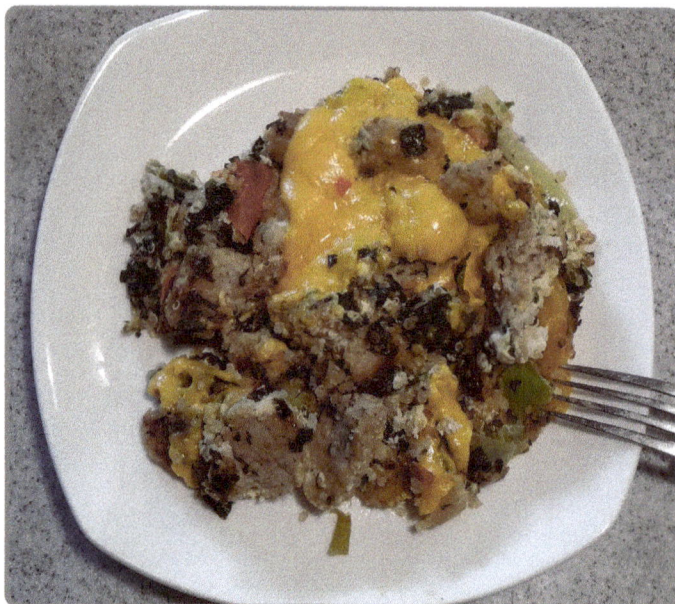

INGREDIENTS

2 tbsp. of cold-pressed organic avocado oil or olive oil

3/4 cup of chopped leeks

3/4 cup of chopped frozen or fresh mixed-color organic bell peppers

6 medium pre-cooked organic free-range chicken or turkey meatballs, quartered (can be a frozen product or made fresh beforehand)

3/4 cup of chopped frozen or fresh organic spinach

1 cup of cooked quinoa

1/2 cup of pasteurized organic egg whites (or 4 fresh organic egg whites)

4 slices of non-dairy cheddar cheese (Almond, soy, etc.)

1/3 tsp. salt

1/4 tsp. black pepper

PREPARATION

Put oil in an 8-inch, nonstick frying pan and heat on medium for 1 minute, then add onions. Cook for 3 minutes on medium-high heat. Add peppers, salt, and pepper and cook for 3 minutes. Add meatball pieces and cook for 3 minutes. Add spinach and cook for 3 minutes. Add cooked quinoa and cook for 2 minutes. Add egg white and cover pan with lid. Cook on medium-low heat until the egg whites are firm. Add cheese and cover. Turn heat off and let sit until cheese melts before serving.

Ingredients replaced: whole eggs, dairy-based cheese, butter, pork bacon, and excessive salt

Chicken and Waffle

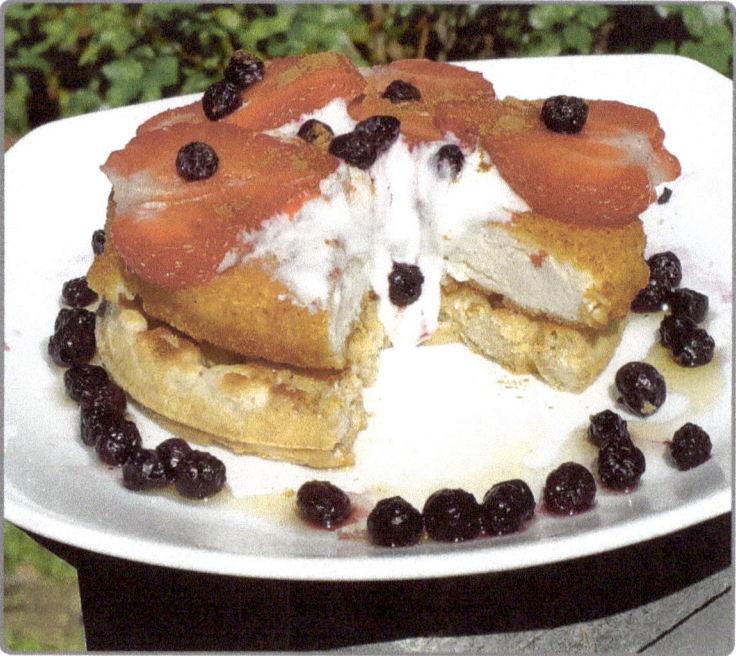

INGREDIENTS

1 tsp. of organic, cold-pressed olive oil

1 pre-cooked, breaded organic chicken patty

1 whole-wheat frozen waffle (can be multi-grain or gluten-free)

1 tsp. of honey

1 tbsp. of non-dairy sour cream

1/2 tsp. of cinnamon

1 large organic strawberry, sliced (can be frozen)

1/4 cup of organic blueberries (can be frozen)

PREPARATION

Place oil in non-stick, 6-inch frying pan and heat for 1 minute on medium heat. Place frozen chicken patty into ceramic pan. Cook on both sides until browned.

Toast waffle. Place waffle in dish and put honey evenly on top. Place chicken patty on top, and spread sour cream on top of patty. Place strawberries and blueberries on top and to the side. Sprinkle top with cinnamon.

Ingredients replaced: butter and dairy sour cream

Bellini Italian Breakfast Pastina

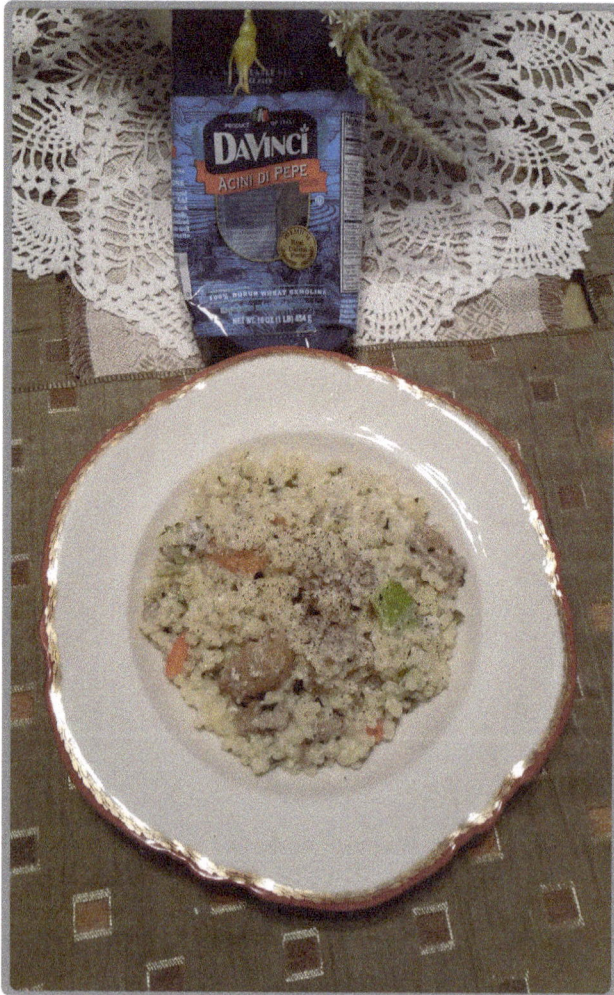

INGREDIENTS

1 tbsp. of extra-virgin cold-pressed olive oil

1/2 cup of chopped organic leeks

1/2 cup of mixed colored organic bell peppers

1/2 cup of organic spinach

1/2 cup of pearl onions

1 cup of chopped, pre-cooked chicken Italian sausage or turkey meatballs.

1 cup of filtered water

1/2 cup of organic egg whites

1 cup of low-sodium chicken broth

2 tbsp. of Italian seasoning

1 tsp. of salt

1/2 tsp. of pepper.

1 pound of Pastina, also known as Acini Di Pepe or orzo pasta

1 tbsp. of non-dairy butter substitute

Non-dairy sour cream as a topping (if desired)

PREPARATION

Place olive oil in a 3-quart pan and heat for 1 minute. Add leeks, peppers, and spinach and cook for 5 minutes. Add chopped sausage or meatballs and cook for 5 minutes. Remove from pan and place on a dish.

Boil 3 cups of water and 2 cups of chicken broth in a pot; add salt, pepper, and pasta. Cook, constantly stirring, until the pasta absorbs the water. If water and broth is cooked away and pasta is still not cooked (taste for hardness), add a little more chicken broth. While still simmering, add all the ingredients you first cooked. Stir in egg whites, place lid on pot, and cook on low heat for 5 minutes, constantly stirring. When done, stir in butter substitute. Plate and garnish with a spoonful of non-dairy sour cream.

Ingredients replaced: butter, dairy sour cream, pork sausage, and whole eggs

Smoothie

INGREDIENTS

1 large organic strawberry, sliced (fresh or frozen)

1/4 cup of organic blueberries (fresh or frozen)

8 oz. of coconut or almond vanilla-flavored milk

1/2 cup of almond or coconut yogurt

1 tbsp. of almond butter

PREPARATION

Pour the almond milk into a blender with strawberry and blueberries. Blend for 10 seconds, then add almond butter and yogurt. Blend to liquefy.

Ingredients replaced: whole milk, peanut butter, and dairy yogurt

Lunch or Dinner

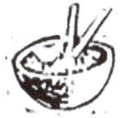

The following recipes can be prepared for lunch or dinner. I recommend that dinner meals contain fewer carbohydrates than lunch as a way of avoiding weight gain.

Manastada (Zuppa di Scarola e Fagioli)

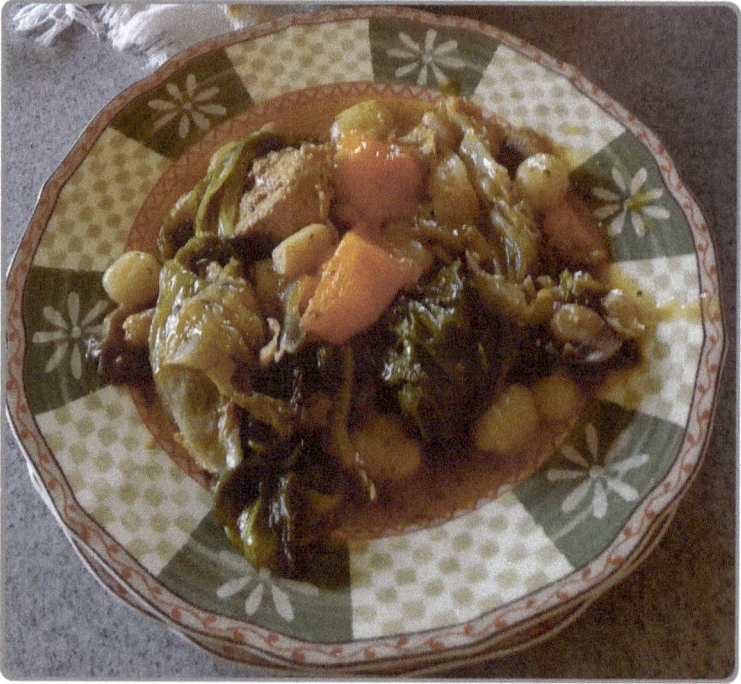

My family called this dish "*manastada*" and I added a few more ingredients to the original to make it a complete meal in one pan. This is my version of an Italian healthy meal by my great-grandfather, Barto Bellini.

INGREDIENTS

3 tbsp. of cold-pressed organic olive oil

Italian chicken sausages (about 3 pounds), with casings removed

1 cup of chopped organic onion

1 cup of sliced organic mushrooms

1 tbsp. of minced organic garlic

1/2 tsp. of dried crushed red pepper

1 large head of organic escarole, chopped (about 10 cups)

3/4 cup of dry white wine

2 15-oz. cans of cannellini beans, rinsed and drained

3 cups of organic chicken stock

Non-dairy Parmesan cheese (optional)

4 large, yellow organic tomatoes

12 oz. of potato gnocchi (dried or refrigerated, preferably whole-wheat)

PREPARATION

Heat oil in heavy, large pot over medium-high heat. Working in batches, sauté sausage until cooked through, breaking up with back of spoon, about 6 minutes per batch. Using slotted spoon, transfer sausage to bowl, leaving drippings in pot.

Reduce heat to medium; add onion to pot and sauté until translucent, about 5 minutes. Add mushrooms and sauté 1 minute. Mix in garlic and crushed red pepper. Add beans and cook for 5 minutes, then add chicken broth and heat to a simmer. Add uncooked gnocchi and cook for 5 minutes, then add escarole and sauté until wilted, about 2 minutes. Add wine and cook 2 minutes. Add cooked sausage and simmer 10 minutes to blend flavors. Season to taste with salt and pepper. Transfer to large bowl. Top with grated Parmesan, if desired.

Ingredients replaced: dairy cheese and pork sausage

Turkey Wellington with Phyllo Pastry Dough

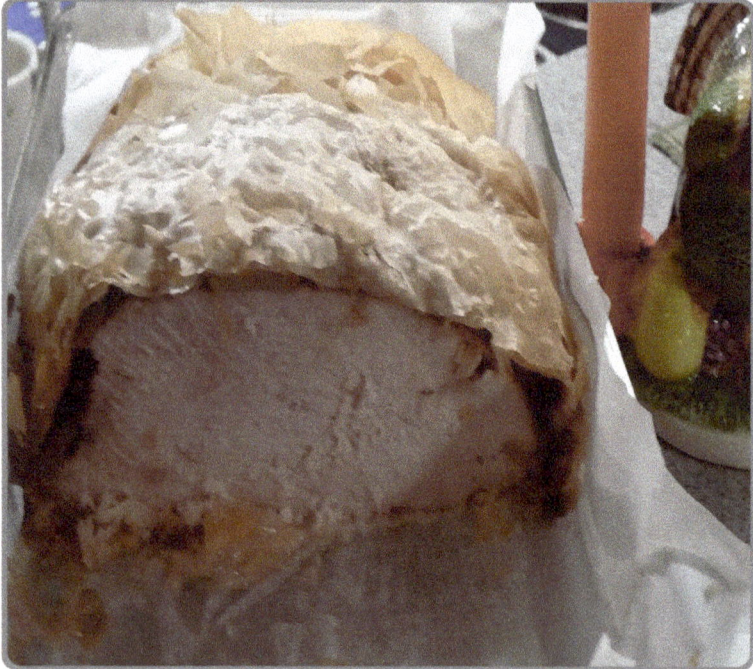

INGREDIENTS

1 whole pre-cooked organic turkey breast (size determined by how many you want to serve)

1 large package of Phyllo pastry dough

1 cup of organic mushrooms, either fresh or from a jar

1 large onion (diced)

2 tbsp. of dried basil

1/4 cup of dried organic tomatoes packed in olive oil (from a jar or fresh)

1 tbsp. extra-virgin cold-pressed olive oil

1 tsp. of salt

1 tsp. of pepper

1/4 cup of white wine

1 large roll of cooking parchment paper

2 tsp. of olive oil

PREPARATION

In a frying pan, heat olive oil for 1 minute on medium-high heat. Then add onion and sauté for 3 minutes. Add tomatoes and cook for another 3 minutes. Add mushrooms, basil, salt, and pepper and cook for 3 minutes. Add wine and cook until wine is mostly evaporated; place to the side.

Line a glass roasting dish with parchment paper (be sure the paper extends from sides of pan to wrap completely around the turkey breast) and rub bottom of paper with olive oil. Place the Phyllo dough on parchment paper followed by the turkey breast. Then add the ingredients previously cooked on top of the turkey breast until top is completely covered. Place the rest of the Phyllo dough on top of turkey breast and seal the sides to bottom dough. Bring the parchment paper from bottom of pan and seal on top so the turkey breast is completely sealed. Place in pre-heated oven of 375° degrees for 45 minutes. Open top of parchment paper to be sure the dough is browned; if not yet browned, continue to cook until it is golden brown. When browned, remove from oven.

Ingredients replaced: Beef roast

Mixed Seafood Cioppino

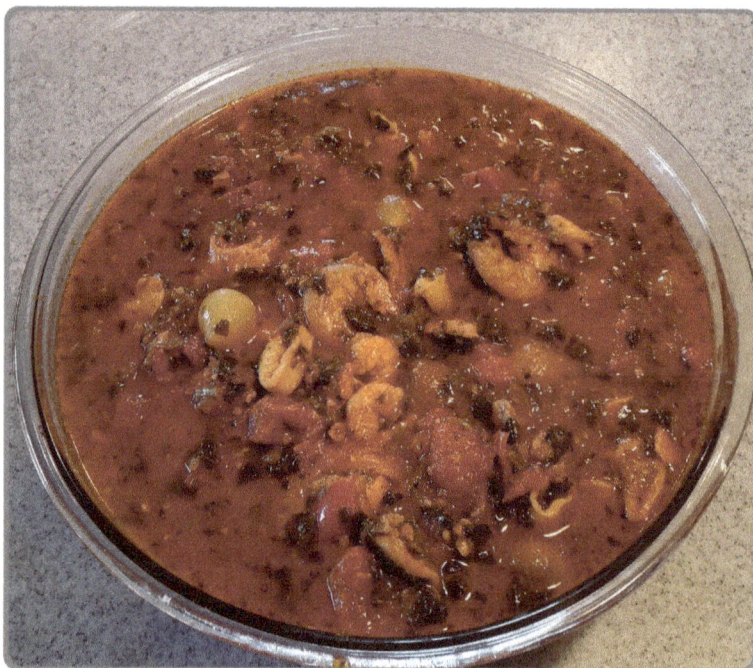

(People with shellfish allergies should substitute only fish in this recipe)

INGREDIENTS

1 package of mixed, wild-caught frozen seafood

1 lb. of wild-caught salmon

2 tbsp. of extra-virgin olive oil

1 cup of spinach

1 bottle of clam juice

1 container of chopped clams

1 tbsp. of chopped organic garlic

1 tsp. of chipotle peppers

4 tbsp. of Italian seasoning

1/2 cup of red wine

2 cups of tomato sauce

5 large Roma tomatoes

1 tsp. of salt

1/2 tsp. of black pepper

PREPARATION

Heat olive oil in a 12-inch frying pan for 1 minute on medium-high. Place seafood into pan and add garlic, salt, and black pepper and cook for 3 minutes. Then add 2 tbsp. of Italian seasoning and cook for 2 minutes, stirring every minute or so until evenly cooked. Remove fish from pan but leave in the leftover oil. Add chopped Roma tomatoes, spinach, salt, black pepper, and remaining Italian seasoning to pan. Cook for 3 minutes and add tomato sauce, clams, and clam juice. Cook for another 3 minutes. Return the seafood to the pan and add the chipotle pepper. Cook for 5 minutes on medium heat. Add red wine and simmer for 3 minutes.

Linguini with Anchovy or Clam Sauce

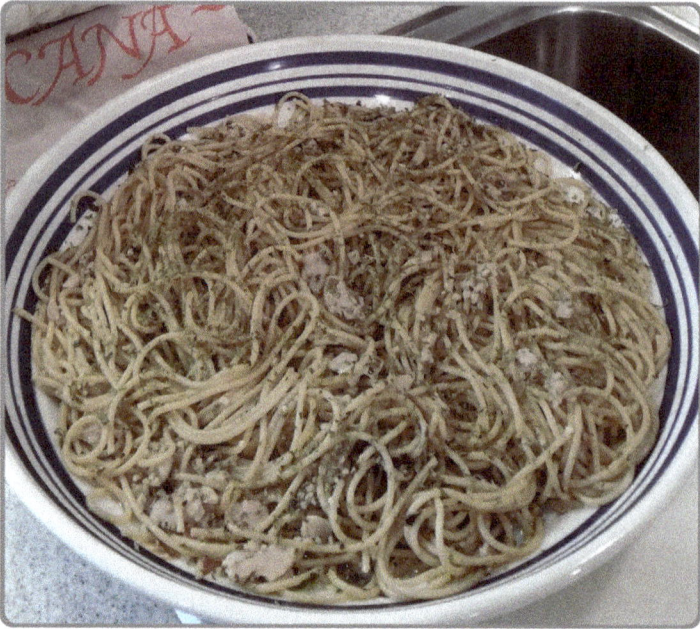

INGREDIENTS

4 tbsp. of extra-virgin cold-pressed olive oil

10 anchovy filets (1 tin) if making anchovy sauce

2 tbsp. of minced garlic

1 tbsp. of dried parsley

12 oz. of chopped clams if making clam sauce

8 oz. of clam juice if making clam sauce

1/4 cup of white wine

1 lb. of linguini, boiled until al dente.

PREPARATION

Place olive oil in a 12-inch frying pan on medium heat for 1 minute and then add anchovies and cook until dissolved. Add the garlic and cook for 3 minutes. Add the white wine and cook for

3 minutes. Add the cooked pasta to the sauce and cook for an additional 3 minutes.

To make the clam sauce follow the above instructions and after adding wine add clam juice and clams. Add basil and cook for 5 minutes, then add pasta as above.

Turkey or Chicken Meatballs

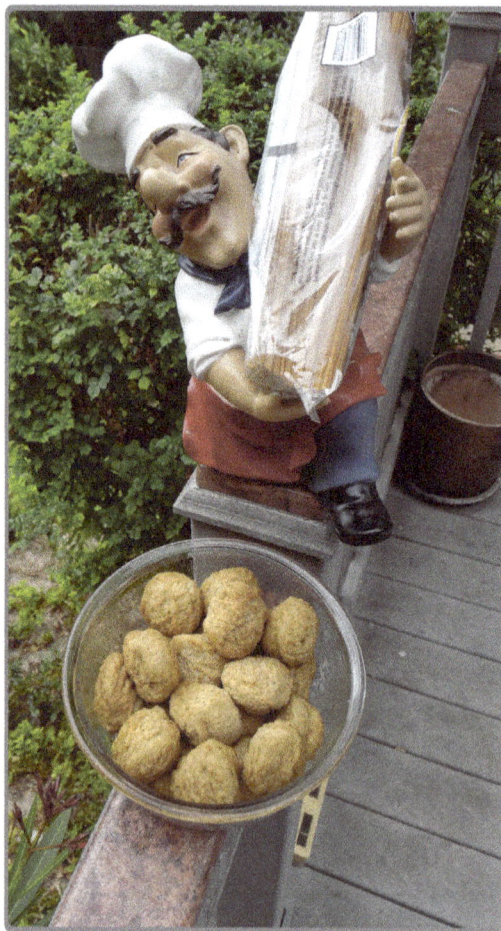

INGREDIENTS

1 lb. of chicken or turkey breast meat

1/4 cup of extra-virgin cold-pressed olive oil

1 tbsp. of dried granulated garlic

4 uncooked organic egg whites

1/2 cup of chopped white onions

1/2 cup of seasoned bread crumbs (No chemicals for preservatives if purchased. To make your own, toast whole wheat bread, grate, and add Italian seasoning.)

1/4 cup of chicken broth

1 tbsp. of dried basil flakes

2 tbsp. of non-dairy Parmesan cheese

1 tbsp. of parsley flakes

PREPARATION

Add meat and 2/3 of olive oil to a large bowl; mix. Add egg whites and mix. Add garlic, white onions, basil, and parsley and continue mixing. Add in breadcrumbs and cheese and mix. Then add chicken broth until the mix is the right consistency to shape the meatballs so they are firm.

Use remaining 1/3 of olive oil to lightly coat bottom of frying pan or baking tray, and then place meatballs in frying pan on medium heat and cook till brown on all sides. Be sure they are cooked through by using a meat thermometer or cut one in half to check the center. (You can also bake on a baking tray at 375° until done.)

Stuffed Bell Peppers

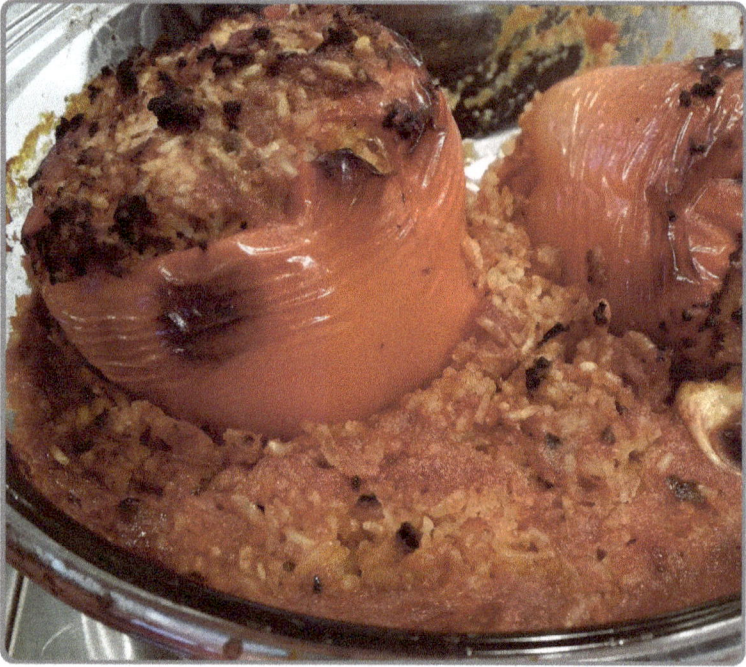

INGREDIENTS

3 large organic bell peppers (any color)

4 cups of cooked brown rice

2 cups of ground, cooked Italian sausage

1 tbsp. of chopped organic garlic

3 cups of tomato sauce

1 tsp. of salt

1/2 tsp. of black pepper

2 tbsp. of organic cold-pressed olive oil

1 medium chopped onion

1/4 cup of shredded almond mozzarella cheese

PREPARATION

In a pan, heat oil and garlic over medium heat for 3 minutes. Add onions and cook for 3 minutes. Add sausage and cook for 5 minutes. Add salt, pepper, rice, and 2 cups of tomato sauce. Cook for 5 minutes.

Core peppers and place the cooked ingredients inside. Place upright in a baking dish with remaining tomato sauce and bake at 375° for 25 minutes. Top pepper with cheese and allow melting for an additional 5 minutes before removing from oven.

Ingredients replaced: white rice, ground beef, and dairy mozzarella cheese

Pasta Con Sarde—Cefalu Style Sicilian Pasta and Sardines

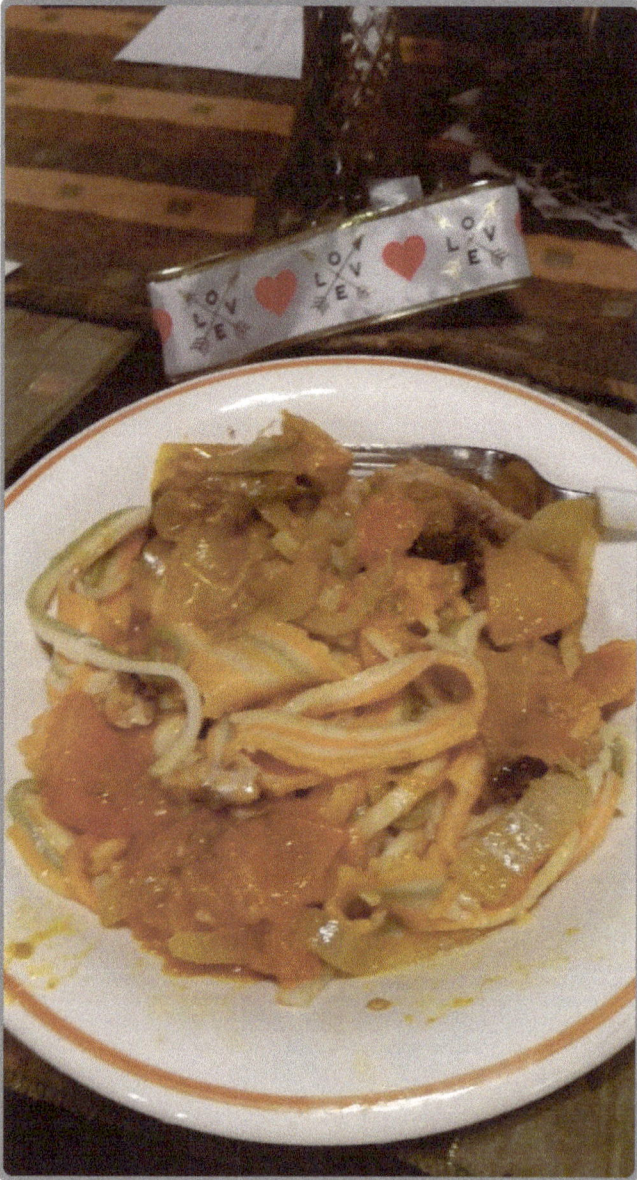

(My special occasion dish)

INGREDIENTS

2 tbsp. of organic extra-virgin olive oil

2 oz. of flat anchovies packed in olive oil

1 large onion, chopped

1 fennel (bulb and stems)

2 tbsp. of powdered fennel

5 large yellow tomatoes, diced

4 tbsp. of yellow raisins

8 medium-sized fresh wild-caught sardines or 2 pre-packaged containers of sardines, preferably in a glass jar, with both jars totaling no less than 8 sardines.

1/2 cup of white wine

1/2 cup of low-salt vegetable broth

1 lb. of fusilli or ribbon pasta

1/2 cup of baked bread crumbs mixed with Italian spice seasoning

PREPARATION

In a 12-inch frying pan, heat olive oil on medium heat for 1 minute and then add anchovies. Cook anchovies until they dissolve, then add the onion. When the onion is browned, add the wine and cook for 2 minutes. Add broth and simmer for 2 minutes. Add chopped fresh fennel and cook for 5 minutes. Add yellow tomatoes and powdered fennel. Cook for 5 minutes on medium heat. Then add yellow raisins and cook for 3 minutes. Last, add the sardines and cook for 5 minutes. Let sit after heat is turned off.

Boil pasta and place in a dish that has been coated with sauce. Pour half the sauce on the pasta and mix thoroughly. Place the remaining sauce on the pasta. Sprinkle the breadcrumbs on top of the pasta just before serving.

Pizza Gana—Easter Pizza Pie

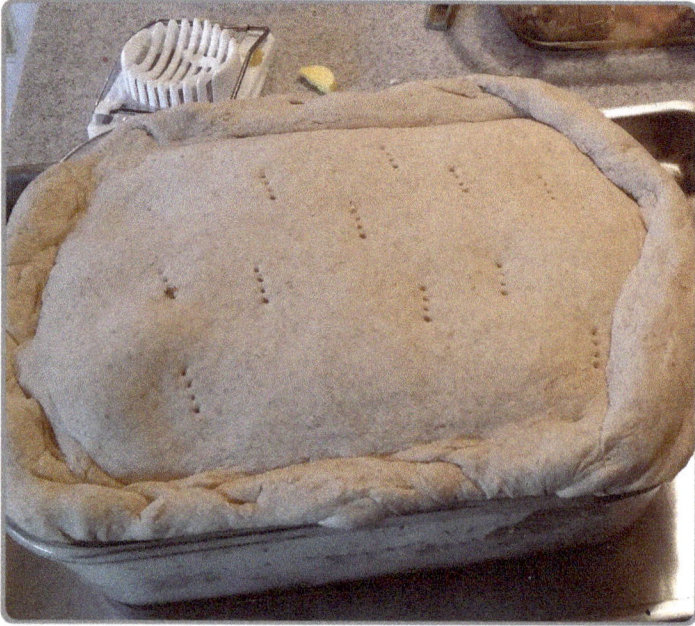

(This is a once-a-year dish that my family makes each Easter.)

INGREDIENTS

2 pre-made whole-wheat pizza dough rounds, which can be purchased in a pizza restaurant or at the supermarket

1 package of extra-firm organic tofu

1 package of organic firm tofu

4 tbsp. of organic cold-pressed olive oil

3/4 cup of organic egg whites

4 tbsp. of parsley flakes

1 tsp. of salt

1/2 tsp. of black pepper

3 tbsp. of grated non-dairy Parmesan cheese

1/2 pound of turkey bacon

1 pound of organic chicken Italian sausage, pre-cooked

10 pre-cooked organic turkey meatballs

8 slices of non-dairy mozzarella cheese (almond or soy)

1/2 cup of shredded non-dairy mozzarella almond cheese

8 hard-boiled organic eggs, whites only (discard yolks)

PREPARATION

Mix both packages of tofu in a large mixing bowl with 3 tbsp. of olive oil, half of the egg whites, parsley, salt, pepper, Parmesan cheese, and shredded mozzarella cheese. Set to side. Cook bacon in frying pan till crisp. Cook sausage and meatballs if raw.

Roll out one round of dough after first allowing it to rise for about an hour. In a glass baking dish, coat the bottom and sides with olive oil and then place the dough in the pan so it covers the bottom and sides. Place in the oven at 400 degrees until slightly browned.

Remove from oven and alternate layers of bacon, tofu blend, sausage, 1/2 of the hard-boiled egg whites, 4 slices of mozzarella, tofu blend, sliced meat balls, remaining hard-boiled egg whites, tofu blend, and 4 mozzarella slices.

Roll out the remaining dough round and place it on top; seal the sides to the bottom dough. Coat with olive oil and place in the oven on top of a cooking pan for about 45 minutes. When top layer of dough starts to brown after about 25 minutes, cover with parchment so it won't burn. When sides of the pan start bubbling, it's done. Remove from oven and allow cooling before serving.

Ingredients replaced: ricotta cheese, mozzarella cheese, whole eggs with yolks, pork meats

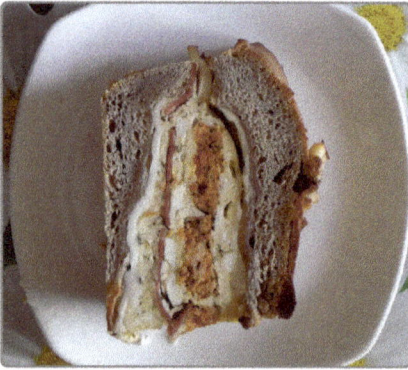

Finished Slice of Pizza Gana:

Note for your lasagna test: Make lasagna using the same Ricotta substitute recipe used above. Use meatballs, sausage, and all the same cheeses as above. Use boiled whole-wheat noodles. Create your own lasagna from this and the other recipes in this book, (i.e., eggplant pasta, etc.). Consider how creative you have become in your alternative thinking.

Salmon Patties with Raspberry-Jalapeno Mustard Sauce, Quinoa, and Broccoli Florets

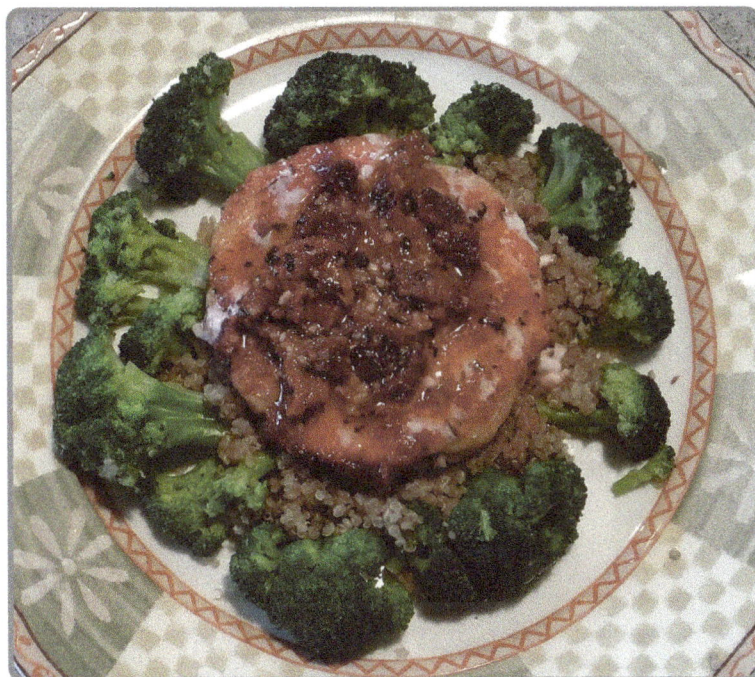

INGREDIENTS

4 wild-caught frozen or fresh salmon patties

1 tbsp. of extra-virgin cold-pressed olive oil

1 tbsp. of chopped organic garlic

1/4 cup of dried organic tomatoes

1 tbsp. of dried basil

4 tsp. of raspberry jalapeno mustard

1/4 cup of white wine

1 cup of broccoli florets (frozen or fresh)

1 cup of previously cooked quinoa (follow directions on quinoa package for cooking—you may also add sautéed chopped celery and onion to quinoa when it is finished cooking.)

PREPARATION

Place olive oil in 12-inch frying pan and heat for one minute. Add garlic, tomatoes, and basil and simmer for 2 minutes, then add wine and continue to cook for another 2 minutes. Place 4 salmon patties on top of cooked mixture and spread 1 tsp. of mustard on top of each patty. Cook for 2 minutes and then turn over salmon patties. Cook for 4 minutes and turn over again. Put top on pan and cook for 4 minutes on medium-low heat.

Spread cooked quinoa on a plate. Put salmon patties on top and steamed broccoli around the edges. Spoon out the mixture of ingredients in the pan on top of salmon patties and on broccoli.

Chicken Parmigianino

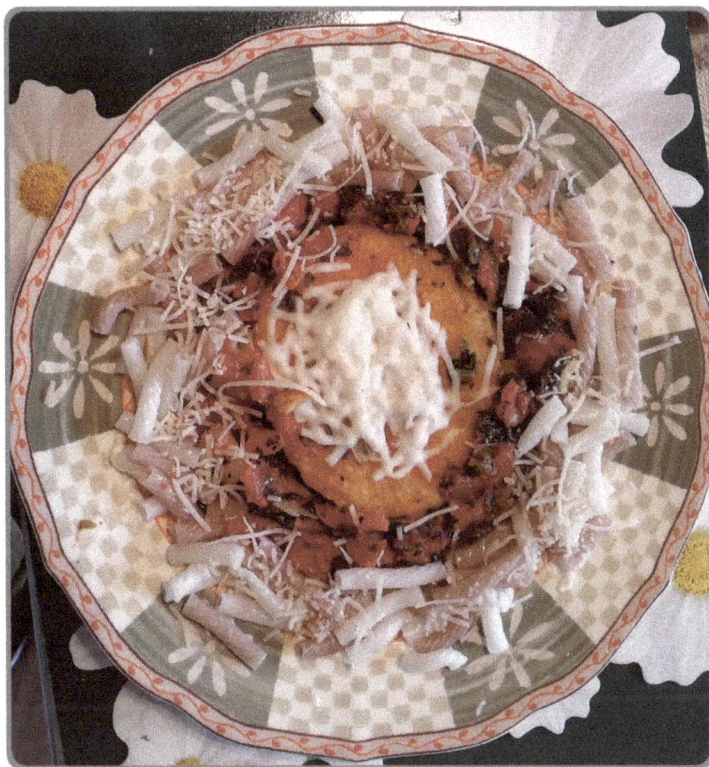

INGREDIENTS

4 breaded, pre-cooked organic chicken patties

2 tbsp. of organic olive oil

1 jar of organic tomato sauce

4 chopped Roma tomatoes

1 clove of garlic

1 cup of organic fresh or frozen spinach

1 cup of sliced organic mushrooms

4 slices of almond organic mozzarella cheese

1/4 cup of dried tomatoes packed in olive oil

4 tbsp. of dried basil

1/4 cup of red wine

3 tbsp. of chopped dried parsley

PREPARATION

In a 12-inch frying pan place olive oil and sauté the garlic that has all been chopped in half. When brown, add mushrooms, dried tomatoes, basil, and parsley and cook on medium heat for 5 minutes. Add chopped tomatoes and cook for 4 minutes. Then add tomato sauce and red wine and cook for 8 minutes. Remove from pan and put in a serving dish. Place 4 chicken patties in pan and brown on both sides in the remaining oil. When brown, add in all the cooked ingredients and simmer for 10 minutes on low heat. Place cheese on top of each patty, turn off heat, and let stand until cheese is melted before serving. Serve alone or with pasta.

Chinese Stir-Fry with Edamame Noodles and Salmon

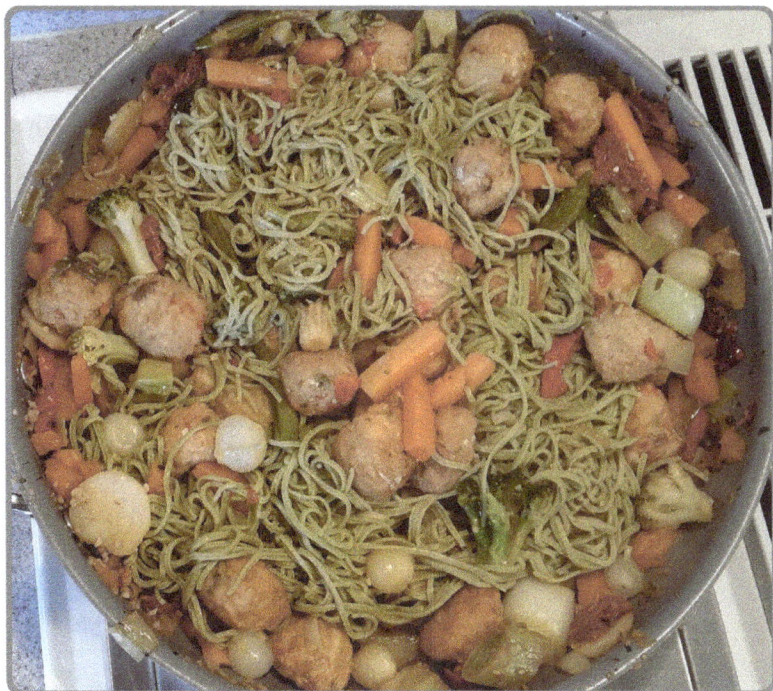

INGREDIENTS

3 tsp. of toasted sesame oil (or avocado oil with 1 tsp. of soy sauce)

1 lb. of fresh or pre-cooked salmon (can also be frozen patties)

1/2 cup of vegetable broth

1/3 cup of leeks

1/2 cup of pearl onions

1/2 cup of dried tomatoes

4 tbsp. of crushed garlic

3/4 cup of broccoli, frozen or fresh

1/2 cup of sliced mushrooms

1/2 lb. green edamame thin spaghetti noodles

3/4 cup of julienne carrots

1/4 cup of white wine

1 1/2 tbsp. of salt (use 1 tbsp. for pasta water)

PREPARATION

Add oil and garlic in a 12-inch pan and heat for 1 minute. Add broth. Place salmon in pan and cook until done, checking the center for color or using a thermometer. Remove salmon and chop into quarter-inch size pieces and leave oil and juices in pan. Add wine and simmer 1 minute. Add leeks, pearl onions, tomatoes, mushrooms, carrots, and broccoli. Cook with added salt for 5 minutes or until tender.

Boil pasta with 1 tbsp. salt in water and cook until al dente (it cooks fast, so taste often).

Chicken and White Bean Chili

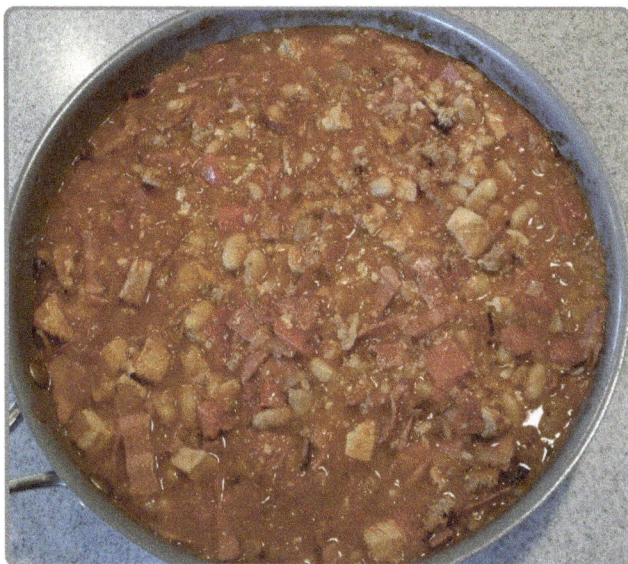

INGREDIENTS

1 can of great northern white beans

3 tbsp. of extra-virgin olive oil

1 lb. of ground chicken or turkey

1/2 lb. of chicken strips

1 medium white onion

1 yellow bell pepper

2 tsp. of salt

1 tsp. of white or black pepper

2 tsp. of fennel seed

4 medium yellow tomatoes (or red tomatoes if desired), cubed

1/2 cup of low-sodium chicken broth

1/4 cup of white wine

1/2 cup of shredded almond mozzarella cheese

PREPARATION

In a 12-inch ceramic frying pan, place the olive oil, chopped onions, and chopped yellow pepper; sauté until soft and then add salt and pepper. Add ground chicken, fennel seeds, and 1-inch chicken strips. Cook until meat is browned and then de-glaze with the white wine. Add great northern white beans and cook until they are done, about 5 to 10 minutes. Add chicken broth and cubed yellow tomatoes. Cook until thick and then turn off heat. Sprinkle the top of the chili with mozzarella cheese and place cover on frying pan. When the cheese is melted, it's ready to eat.

Ingredients replaced: Ground beef, beef cubes, and dairy-based cheese

Pasta with Eggplant

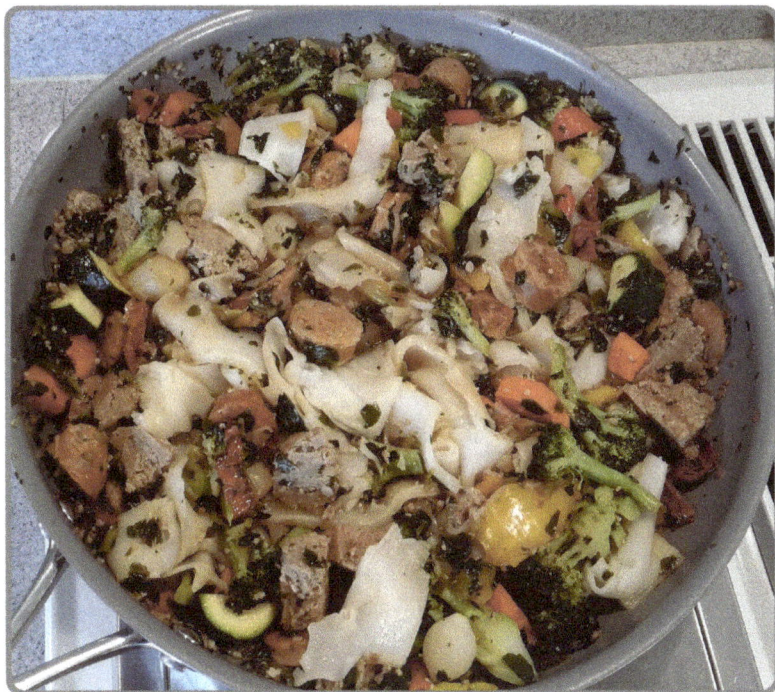

INGREDIENTS

5 large, red organic cubed tomatoes

2 tbsp. of organic olive oil

3 tbsp. chopped organic garlic

1/3 cup of dried tomatoes packed in olive oil

1 lb. of Chinese or Japanese organic eggplant, cubed

4 organic scallions, chopped

1/4 cup of white wine

1/4 cup of low-sodium chicken broth

1/4 cup of Greek olives

1/2 lb. of Italian sausage

1/2 lb. of Pantacce pasta (or 2-inch broken pieces of lasagna noodles)

Shredded or grated Parmigianino cheese

PREPARATION

Heat olive oil 1 minute on medium heat. Add garlic, scallions, and dried tomatoes and cook for 3 minutes. Add eggplant and cook for 5 minutes or until tender. Add white wine and cook for 3 minutes, then add chicken broth with olives and cook for an additional 3 minutes. Add tomatoes and simmer on medium-low heat for 10 minutes. Add in cooked pasta and cook and stir for 3 minutes. Sprinkle with cheese and serve.

Chicken or Turkey Breast Italian Sausage

NOTE: If you take the ingredients to some meat departments in a grocery store, that make sausage, they may grind it and put it in casings for you if you buy the chicken breasts in their store.

INGREDIENTS

10 lbs. ground or whole organic chicken or turkey breast

2 oz. of fennel seed

1/2 oz. of crushed red pepper

2 oz. of salt

2 1/2 oz. of paprika

1 cup of olive oil and 2 cups of low-sodium chicken broth (if using pork, replace broth with water)

PREPARATION

If meat is ground, mix all ingredients together in a bowl. If you have whole breast meat, have it ground either in your own machine or in a grocery store. As mentioned, some grocery stores will make the sausage for you as long as you take them all the ingredients and buy your meat there.

To cook, place in a frying pan with 3 tbsp. of olive oil and about ¼ inch of water. Place on low heat and cook until water evaporates and the sausage sizzles and browns.

Ingredients replaced: Pork butt

Bellini's Homemade Pasta Sauce

When my cousin Johnny heard I was adding recipes to this book, he reminded me that when he was a kid, he really enjoyed eating pasta at our home. Back then, the sauce was filled with large amounts and varieties of red meats, which were not truly found in Italian cooking in Italy. Many people don't know this, but much cooking in this country is not truly ancestral. Instead, it has changed due to the availability of cheap red meat, thereby leading to our country's weigh problems. The recipe below is a prime example of how to replace unhealthy meats with healthier alternatives.

INGREDIENTS

8 large organic Roma diced tomatoes

3 tbsp. of extra-virgin olive oil

10 cloves of organic garlic, chopped

1/2 cup of organic low-salt chicken broth

1 lb. of organic chicken sausage (pre-cooked, frozen or fresh)

8 organic turkey meatballs (pre-cooked, frozen or fresh)

12 oz. of tomato sauce

4 tbsp. of dried basil

2 tbsp. of oregano

1/2 cup of fresh organic basil leaves

1/2 a chopped onion

1/2 cup of chopped organic spinach

1/2 cup of organic diced bell peppers multi colored

1 oz. of non-dairy Parmesan cheese

1/4 of cup red wine

PREPARATION

Place the olive oil in a 12-inch pan and heat for 1 minute on medium heat. Add garlic, onion, and peppers; simmer until lightly brown, constantly stirring. Remove garlic and onions, leaving the oil. Then add all the meatballs and cook until browned. Remove the meatballs and place the sausage in the pan. Add 1/4 cup of chicken broth and 1/4 cup of water and cook until done, approximately 10 minutes.

Return meatballs, garlic, and onions to pan, and add the diced tomatoes, dried basil, and oregano seasoning. Cook for 5 minutes on medium heat and then add in the spinach. Cook for 5 minutes. When the tomatoes are cooked soft, add in the tomato sauce and cook for another 10 minutes on medium-low heat. Add red wine and cook for 3 minutes. Add in the Parmesan cheese and cook for 5 minutes.

Boil your favorite pasta al dente and place pasta in bowl and mix with sauce, leaving enough sauce in pan to put on top of pasta in the individual dish. Some people prefer to put cooked pasta in the saucepan and cook it with the sauce for 3 minutes. This is especially needed when using whole-wheat pasta.

Sprinkle top of pasta with cheese.

Ingredients replaced: Pork sausage, beef meatballs, pork chops, beef cubes, and dairy-based cheese. This quick-cook recipe also has a lower acid and sugar content than overcooked sauces.

Olive Oil Pizza

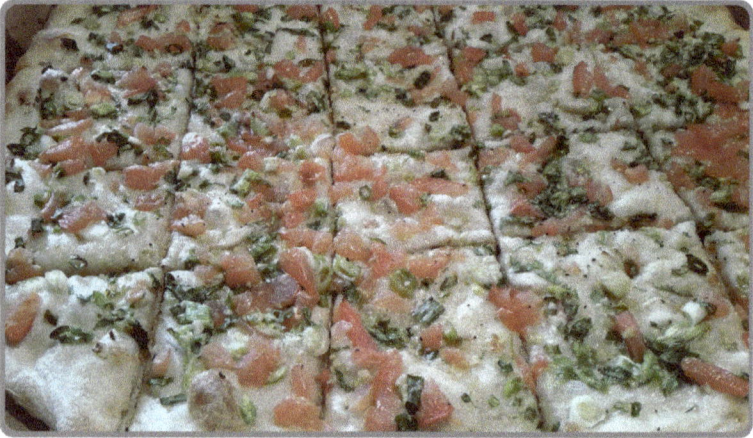

INGREDIENTS

Whole wheat pizza dough

6 large Roma tomatoes, chopped

1/2 cup of chopped garlic

1/4 cup of extra-virgin cold-pressed olive oil

1/2 cup of chopped fresh basil

1/2 cup of chopped scallions

1 tsp. of salt

1 tsp. of pepper

3 tbsp. of non-dairy Parmesan (GO VEGGIE grated Parmesan is my favorite)

PREPARATION

Place in a mixing bowl tomatoes, garlic, 1/4 cup of olive oil, basil, and scallions and mix. Sprinkle on salt and pepper and mix. Place to one side for 15 minutes. After allowing the pizza dough to rise on the counter for 1/2 hour, roll out the pizza dough to about ¼-inch thickness. Brush on top lightly with olive oil. Place in a preheated oven on top of a pizza stone at 400 degrees until pizza dough is slightly brown. Remove from oven, brush on more olive oil, and add the marinated tomato mixture on top of slightly cooked pizza dough and return to the oven for about 10 minutes. Remove from oven, brush edges of pizza with remaining olive oil, and sprinkle with Parmesan.

About the Author

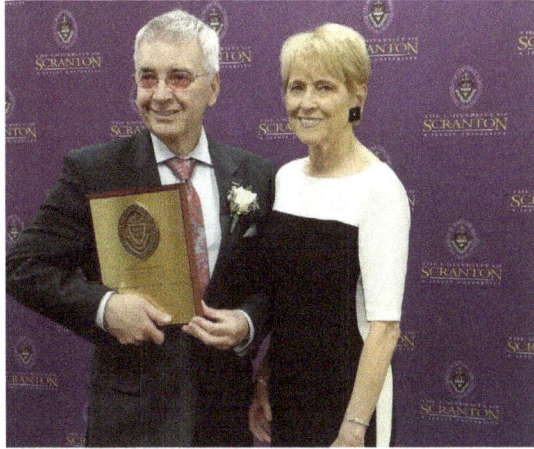

DR. BART P. BILLINGS has been working in the fields of mental health, human services, research and program development, and management for over fifty years. He possesses licenses in clinical

Recieving the Frank O Hara 2016 award at the Universuty of Scranton; highest award the Jesuit University gives. Pictured with my wife, Jeanie.

psychology and marriage and family therapy. He also has past expertise as a certified rehabilitation counselor. He has an extensive background in management and program development and founded the Institute For Occupational Services (IOS).

He was the commanding officer for an Army Reserve general hospital section and has served a total of approximately thirty-four years in the US Army as enlisted and as an officer. His highest military rank was colonel (SCNG-SC medical directorate). In this capacity, he founded and directed The Annual International Military and Civilian Combat Stress Conferences, Prisoner of War Conferences, and the Human Assistance Rapid Response Team (HARRT), which was accepted at the Pentagon in 1997 as a readiness protocol to be implemented military-wide.

Dr. Billings has been a featured guest on HBO's Vice News (previously ABC's Nightline) and U.S. News and World Report. He has been featured on national and international documentaries, TV news shows, and extensive radio shows discussing combat stress. He has given testimony to congressional and state legislative hearings to emphasize the need for better mental health treatment programs for military personnel and their families. These hearings have resulted in multi-million-dollar Department of Defense grants for national research to improve treatment for PTSD and traumatic brain injuries. He is responsible for initiating congressional hearings to provide testimony regarding the relationship between psychiatric medication and increased suicides in the military (available on the Congressional Record).

He served as a member of the Governor's Advisory Board to Patton State Hospital, California, and is also a member of the National Center for Youth Law Medical and Scientific Advisory Board. He oversaw all psychological services for the San Diego District of the California Department of Rehabilitation. He has developed residential treatment programs in substance abuse and alcoholism, as well as human assistance programs for the civilian and military communities. Dr. Billings served as senior faculty at the William Glasser MD Institute for over thirty years and taught classes at the University of San Francisco, University of California Davis, and United States International University, in addition to presenting workshops on counseling and management throughout the United States.

Dr. Billings speaks on health and nutrition with a focus on the psychology of eating. As prior owner and operator of a restaurant for 5 years, he practiced his teachings in the restaurant. During his years of owning this popular restaurant/bar in La Costa California, he met with many retired and active duty veterans who would share their personal issues with combat stress. His work with veterans during their visits to his restaurant was described in an article in the military section of the *North Coast Times*. His recent book, *Invisible Scars—Treating Combat Stress, PTSD Without Medication* addresses more than forty years of work with the residual effects of combat stress on our veterans and their families.

In February 2014, Dr. Billings received the International Human Rights Award from the Citizens Commission on Human Rights (CCHR). Dr. Billings' most recent award, the Frank O'Hara Award, was presented to him on June 3, 2016 from the University of Scranton, where he received his BS and MS degrees. This prestigious award is given for living the Jesuit values of serving others.

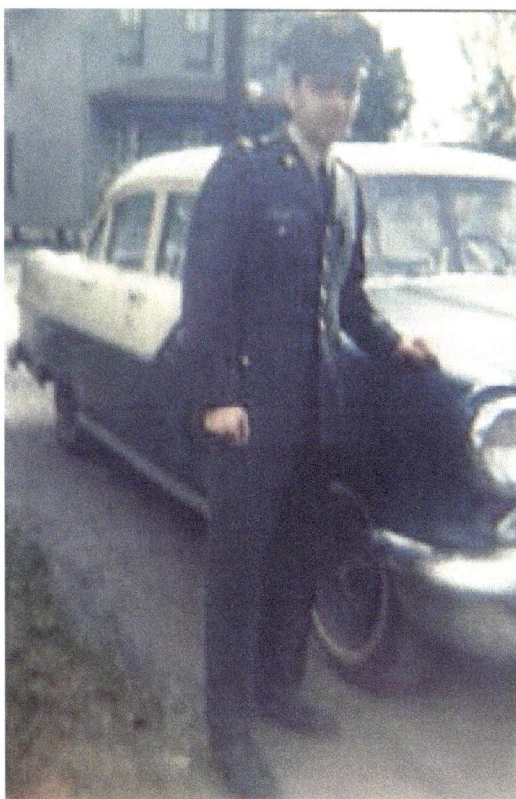

Dr. Billings in 1963 (age 19), with his first car (1955 Pontiac) as a cadet in ROTC at the University of Scranton (Jesuit College in Pennsylvania).

"Medicine cures diseases of the body, wisdom liberates the soul of sufferings."

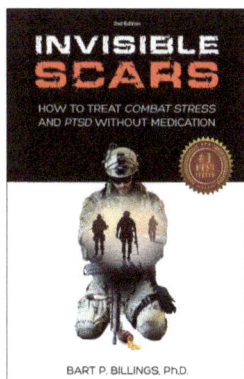

Invisible Scars: How to Treat Combat Stress and PTSD without Medication

INVISIBLE SCARS is the only book specifically addressing and outlining how individuals experiencing combat stress and PTSD are suffering longer and with worsening symptoms, because of the massive use of psychiatric medications. Dr. Billings provides an uncensored description and data showing the dangers involved in taking psychiatric medications, and he explains in clear and concise terms how to work with individuals, without the use of psychiatric medications.

Of the 2.4 million U.S. troops, who have been deployed to Iraq and Afghanistan, 30% return home with post-traumatic stress due to combat related stress and more than 320,000 suffer from traumatic brain injury (TBI). Many more are misdiagnosed or are not diagnosed at all. Troops, who are exposed to PTSD in the form of high levels of stress and anxiety during combat are more likely to withdraw, engage in substance abuse, show signs of depression, or even commit suicide after returning home.

GET THE BOOK THAT VETERANS PEER GROUPS, BOOK CLUBS ARE USING AS A GUIDE TO SAVING LIVES AT: http://bartpbillings.com.

International Combat Stress Conference

This website provides information about the International Combat Stress Conference. Other stress control and debriefing resources including historical information also available here to assist you!

NOTICE: This website is unofficial and contains no classified materials or information.

www.combatstress.bizhosting.com